KT-104-630

Emotional Healing
through
Mindfulness
Meditation

Stories and Meditations
for Women Seeking Wholeness

Barbara Miller Fishman, Ph.D.

Inner Traditions
Rochester, Vermont

Inner Traditions
One Park Street
Rochester, Vermont 05767
www.InnerTraditions.com

Copyright © 2002 by Barbara Miller Fishman, Ph.D.

All rights reserved. No part of this book may be reproduced or utilized in any form or
by any means, electronic or mechanical, including photocopying, recording, or by any
information storage and retrieval system, without permission in writing from the
publisher. The stories in this book are fictional composites. None of the characters in
the stories represent real people, either living or dead.

Library of Congress Cataloging-in-Publication Data
Fishman, Barbara Miller.
  Emotional healing through mindfulness meditation : stories and
  meditations for women seeking wholeness / Barbara Miller
Fishman.
      p. cm.
Includes bibliographical references.
  ISBN 0-89281-998-7
  1. Meditation—Therapeutic use. 2. Women—Mental health.
3. Psychotherapy. I. Title.
  RC489.M43 F54 2002
  616.89'0082—dc21

                                    2002014764

Printed and bound in the United States at Lake Book Manufacturing, Inc

10 9 8 7 6 5 4 3 2 1

Text design and layout by Priscilla Baker
This book was typeset in Berkeley

I dedicate this book to:

My teacher, Shinzen Young, for the simply stated, complex teachings
that led me to discover the subtle unfolding
of a spiritual life;

Alyson Scott, my dear friend, whose penetrating questions
and heartfelt support went a long way toward making the birth
of this book a reality;

Bob Fishman, my husband, for the gift of a miraculous love
that unites us as "two solitudes that protect and border
and salute each other."

Contents

Acknowledgments viii

Foreword ix

Preface xi

Introduction
The Only Way Out Is Through . . . 1

One ∞
How Tanya Found Her Song 12
A Meditation on Finding the Stillness 30

Two ∞
Kate's Loving Addiction 33
A Meditation on Cultivating Awareness 51

Three ∞
Sex, Fantasy, and a Married Woman Named Laura 55
A Meditation on the Thinking Mind 70

Four ∽

Maria   73

A Meditation on Equanimity and the Judging Mind   92

Five ∽

How Nancy Gave Birth to a Healer   95

A Meditation on Seeing through the Lens of Impermanence   116

Six ∽

Strawberries   119

A Meditation on the Nature of Self   128

Seven ∽

Mae Is Changing the World   133

A Meditation on Anger   155

Eight ∽

Harriet's Love Story   159

A Meditation on Loving Kindness   178

Nine ∽

Marcia Wants to Live until She Dies   181

A Meditation on Letting Go   205

Epilogue   208

Notes   215

Bibliography   222

Acknowledgments

I thank the following people for their interest, their readiness to engage, and their support: My three sons and their wives, who read and responded to parts of the manuscript and told me stories about child-rearing that often found their way into the book. Michael Denomme, whose careful and perceptive reading was both supportive and discriminating at the same time. Beth-Ellen Kroope, whose belief in the book came at just the right time. Colleen McCarthy, Judy Erhman, Mary Gregorio, and Ginnie Davidov, who all contributed in the role of readers. Last, I'm thankful to Gretchen Wilson and David Key for spending evenings listening to me read.

Foreword

It's easy to become discouraged when we consider the state of the world, in which violence, injustice, terrorism, and national myopia seem more than ever in ascendance. Yet I find myself strangely optimistic about our global prospects. Below the present surface turbulence, I detect a deep and unprecedented historical movement as yet largely unheralded in the mainstream media. The two most powerful discoveries of all time—the scientific method of the West and the meditative technology of the East—have finally met and are beginning to interact vigorously. It is my belief that they will mate, giving birth to a generation of strange and powerful tools for the benefaction (and perhaps even salvation) of this world.

The book you have before you has arisen from the initial courtship of these two forces. It tells the stories of eight women who overcame enormous challenges. Although the nature of their challenges differed, the basic procedure that allowed them to transmute emotional pain into life energy was the same—a hybrid of Western psychotherapy potentiated with Buddhist mindfulness exercises. By reading their stories you will get a tangible sense of what it means to literally escape *into* pain, as opposed to escaping from it—a truly remarkable notion.

Dr. Barbara Fishman, the author of this book, has been studying Mindfulness Meditation with me for more than fifteen years. Her practice is rigorous and deep. She is part of a growing cadre of psychotherapists who are experimenting with bringing Buddhist mindfulness techniques into the practice of psychotherapy. This work, I believe, represents the first eddy of a tide that will mold the twenty-first century.

SHINZEN YOUNG
DIRECTOR, VIPASSANA SUPPORT INSTITUTE

Preface

We're expecting a major snowstorm as I write these words. Outside, the wind is strangely calm, and the sky is a steely gray. I can feel the tension that comes with an impending storm. It's much like the wind—restless and uneasy. A worrisome thought passes through my mind: Will my husband and I be safe as we travel down the length of the Pennsylvania turnpike later in the day? Fortunately, this little mountain home of ours is a warm and cozy place from which to view the danger outside, so I reassure myself about the capacity of our road crews to manage the icy accumulation; I grow quiet inside and continue to write.

Storms also blow through our psyches. Triggered by trouble in the outside world, perhaps a crash in the stock market or the loss of a loved one, inner turmoil can rage as harshly as any blizzard. And the damage done to us, though of a different sort, can be as great as that of any weather disaster. We suffer less if we have a way of sheltering ourselves, a grounding from which to watch the storms.

The motivation to write *Emotional Healing through Mindfulness Meditation* comes from a lifelong effort to grapple with these internal storms, both in my own life and in those I encounter in my work as a psychotherapist. And the central question has always been, How do we shelter ourselves so that the very protection we need doesn't imprison us within our own defenses, perhaps in the form of a chronic withdrawal or a scowl that threatens harm? Is it possible to feel safe in a way that allows for engaged, open, and loving responses to life?

The wonder is that, at this point in my life, I can answer these questions with a deeply felt "Yes!" It has taken many years to find that answer, though even now I can lose sight of it for periods of time. But I do know a path that can help me find that yes again. I call it a path toward wholeness, and it makes use of both psychotherapy and meditation to heal the emotions.

Like most of us, I've tried many ways to shelter myself from tumultuous emotions. My first attempt was to find shelter *outside,* in the world, through the approval of others and the accumulation of achievements. Both of these felt good—when I got them. But neither one protected me from the storms of uncertainty and loneliness that blew through periodically. Not that I want to negate the effort; approval and achievement brought the esteem of others. It's just that the outcome was ultimately disappointing. The storms still came with almost the same intensity.

I tried to find shelter *inside,* in my own psyche. My first conscious effort to do this was when I tried to read the writings of Sigmund Freud. They piqued my interest, maybe because I was an adolescent and thought they had something to do with sex; however, only the rudiments of his work made any sense at all. Nevertheless, in the years following, I went to school and learned how to think "psychologically." And so I grounded myself in an understanding of emotions—my own and those of others. Even being able to name a personal emotion such as anxiety or sadness helped. Now there was some space between me and my inner turmoil, especially after the emotion faded enough for me to reflect on it.

And I became a psychotherapist, which meant learning more about troublesome emotions right in my own office. I am immensely grateful to those I have worked with over the years; in the best of therapy sessions, both of us gained insight and took steps in our own development.

All the while, life itself taught me to find the shelter that comes with knowing one's way around trouble. Suffering through the emotional turmoil of marital arguments, the loss of parents, and children's illnesses, I learned to expect trouble, and I learned that it held both pain and opportunity. Even in the midst of a raging internal storm, it became important to stay exposed long enough to identify that opportunity.

Then I began to meditate. Now my search for shelter took another leap. Because I could more carefully watch the thoughts and feelings that were part of my emotions, I was able to hear myself think, *I'm lonely,* or *I'm angry,* and I understood that the verb *I am* was a problem. Using that verb, I was so fully identified with my turbulent emotions that there was no space between them and me. I *was* the loneliness. I *was* the anger. Consciously examining emotions helped me to be separate from them—even when in the midst of painful feelings. Meditation was another, more in-the-moment shelter. It gave me the opportunity to try on other emotions and behaviors. And I used what I learned to help others.

Over years of practice, I also came to understand that meditation was more than a method; it was a way of living very close to all experience. With that understanding came great insights. I watched the way my thoughts and feelings arose, revealed themselves, and then disappeared. I saw both their power and their ever changing, ephemeral nature. Even the boundary between myself and others began to thin as I sensed that we are all experiencing that flow. Sometimes, even in the midst of great turmoil, my mind grew quiet, and I rode the storms much like a great sea bird, high up on top of the winds. Here was the more complete, meditative approach to knowing my troublesome emotions— by being in the midst of the raging storm and outside of it at the same time. As it turned out, when trouble blew in, I needed to find not a storm-resistant shelter but, rather, the stillness that is in the eye of the storm. That stillness was my gateway to a path toward wholeness.

While I've practiced psychotherapy for close to forty years, my practice of meditation dates back fifteen years. By the standards of the latter tradition, I'm very much a beginner. So particularly when it comes to meditation, please think of this book as an introduction, and read more about the practice. Also know that, ultimately, it is only through direct experience that true learning can take place.

With this preface as a beginning, I invite you into the world of *Emotional Healing through Mindfulness Meditation.* If you're intrigued, get to know the women whose stories are told here, and watch how they explored the psychological and spiritual dimensions of their lives. You'll see that the women discovered ways to be safe in the midst of their emotional turmoil *without* deadening themselves in the process. They also learned how to be present and excited by life, even as trouble roared.

There are specific, well-trodden steps you can take to explore emotional healing through Mindfulness Meditation; these steps can be followed by anyone who has the determination to do so. Add to this the use of psychological thinking and psychotherapy, and the storms of life hold great opportunities for well-being. I invite you to try the meditations at the end of each chapter to explore your own mind/body process. The effort helps—not as a magical pill that dissolves all trouble, but as a means of discovering the path toward wholeness. On this path, the self becomes more vibrant, peaceful, and loving.

Even so, the world remains a stormy place. Outside, children shoot each other, criminals steal from us, and terrorists blow up our buildings. Inside, emotions such as fear, anger, and despair often swirl. If we watch closely, we also see that inside and outside profoundly influence each other. For example, when terrorists blow up our buildings, we become angry inside. It's also true that when we rage our way through the day, we're likely to create fear and anger outside, in others. If we want peace, we eventually realize that both the outside and inside worlds present us with the same challenge: to discover the stillness within, and from that stillness, to feel compassion for ourselves and all other beings. Acting from the inside to shape the outside, we might very well change our small part of the earth.

Introduction

The Only Way Out
Is Through . . .

In the beginning there were eight women. They came with secrets, things they had never told anyone. One woman confided that she was in an abusive relationship that led her to try to kill herself. Another, whose lover had died precipitously, spoke of grieving so deeply she felt sure she was going crazy. Still another, married and depressed, disclosed her plan to attend her high school reunion after receiving a letter from an old lover.

Then there were eight triumphs, not the happily-ever-after kind, but the experiences of mastery that became turning points in eight lives. It took years for the magic of each story to unfold. And in each case, both of us, therapist and client, devoted the time to meet where it could happen, at the threshold between the external, material world and the intangible world of meaning that lies within.

What makes each woman's story special for me is that it never ended. Long after the telling, bits and pieces of the tales continued to bubble up in my dreams and musings until they developed an existence of their own. Ultimately they became some mixture of the woman's story, our joint effort to expand her freedom within it, and the stories of others caught in the same struggle. So the women you will get to know in this book are both real *and* imaginary, history *and* myth.

For years I knew I had to write about the women but didn't, perhaps because I couldn't yet understand why they were so important to me. Finally I decided not to wait any longer, trusting that whatever there was to be known would emerge as I wrote. But how would I write about the women? What form would I choose? I knew that the linear writing of professional papers would miss much of what made these women distinctive, and so I finally immersed myself in the multilayered nuance of story. That's when I learned why these women were important to me: they were all seeking wholeness. Every one of them was searching for meaning beyond ordinary experience. To do so, they challenged social convention, gender roles, and the limited nature of everyday thinking.

The narratives in *Emotional Healing through Mindfulness Meditation* are *teaching* or *learning* stories (I actually prefer to call them *healing* stories) written in the tradition of Sufi or Zen tales. For this reason, they are punctuated at points when the women had insights that shifted the ground on which they stood, if only a millimeter or two. These insights led them to make choices that freed them from patterned, habitual behavior and moved them forward on their path toward wholeness. However, each story is but one chapter in a woman's life. Will later chapters build on her triumphs? Will the healing ultimately hold? In an important sense, these questions don't matter. What does matter is that at one time in her life, when she needed to, this woman found the courage to directly experience trouble and all the emotions that came with it, and in the process, she was transformed.

Times are good for those who seek wholeness. Teachers are a little more accessible and knowledge from ancient healing traditions is increasingly available. I, for one, have a growing sense of how the awareness I learned to use in psychotherapy can, through the practice of Mindfulness Meditation, emerge as a classical spiritual path. As these two traditions meet, they are transforming each other—and us.

In this sense, *Emotional Healing through Mindfulness Meditation* is a contribution to the forty- or fifty-year-old conversation in the West about the relationship between Buddhist meditation and psychotherapy.[1] In another sense, this is a book about and for women, the consequence of my longing to offer this half of the human race an affirming mirror to see the beauty and the creativity within. Finally, my deepest hope is that any human being—male or female—who is seeking wholeness will find it useful.

THE PATH

The search for wholeness is essentially an individual effort, something a woman pursues in her dreams and musings and while she's washing the dishes. Following the path takes great courage and considerable curiosity, neither of which comes from psychotherapy or meditation; these traditions are simply the context within which the effort takes place. As it turns out, courage and curiosity are qualities of the seeker herself. The woman brings them to the effort. And because she's at her growing edge, life is out of the ordinary, creative, and once in a while, quite miraculous.

I was intrigued to realize that all eight women shared certain experiences in their search for wholeness. For instance, every one of them began her life as an outsider; whether because of race, class, or a quirk of mind, she didn't belong. It was an isolating experience that, from time to time, caused most of them to scream for relief. But this alone wasn't enough to put them on the path toward wholeness.

All eight women were also in serious trouble when I met them; one woman felt the alienation that comes with being labeled crazy, another the despair that can accompany metastatic cancer. They came very close to death's door or, symbolically, to the end of a phase of their lives. This, too, wasn't enough to set them on the path toward wholeness.

The women found the path only when they discovered the will, the determination to meet their trouble head on. This commitment came with a heavy price. If they wanted to truly live, they had to penetrate the inner turmoil that comes with trouble, be it shame, despair, or any one of a number of difficult emotions. At the same time, they had no idea where this would lead them.

When the women were ready, perhaps sufficiently loosened from everyday thinking, they had experiences of insight, the *ah-ha* that emerges from deep inside when things fit together and one transcends the para-doxical, the ungraspable in life. These were experiences of holistic know-ing. Now the women had some hint of where the search would take them.

With time, the path offered gifts. Emotions that once raged became quiet. The women felt at peace with themselves; they had more energy for life. Talents emerged. Most intriguing, the women began to give back to others the very gifts they had received. One woman offered it through music, another through healing, and all had a greater capacity for com-passion. People were drawn to them; they were distinctive, extraordi-nary. Slowly, in their own small ways, they related to others with the kind of love that can bring peace to our world.

And I understood that, having learned how to navigate the path to-ward wholeness, they would make it a way of life.

PSYCHOTHERAPY AND MINDFULNESS MEDITATION

Many different kinds of human journeys take place in the office of a psychotherapist. Sometimes it's where people struggle with serious per-sonal problems such as mental illness or where healthy families try to figure out how to raise healthy children. More rarely, the therapist finds a seeker sitting before her. Then the challenge is to create a threshold between the material world and the symbolic world wherein both thera-pist and client can explore the unknown. The path is psychological and spiritual, echoing the efforts of healers in other traditions and other times. It is also political, in the sense that it opens the doors of compassion, and along with that comes a need to mend the world.

I used the tools of psychotherapy to help each woman explore her story, touch feelings she may have denied or repressed, and name the predominant themes or patterns that shaped her life. We also traced the roots of those themes across generations. Then we worked with her story until it was less driven by old patterns and more aligned with who she wanted to be. Getting to know the emotions that drove the old patterns, the women felt more grounded. In these ways, psycho-therapy offered each woman a way to lead the examined life.

Being a student of Buddhist Meditation, I also used this ancient discipline. Sometimes a woman happened upon the meditative experience on her own in the course of her suffering. I taught others the basics of the skill. And so they all eventually learned how to train the powerful microscope that is meditation on the mind/body process, which means they began to observe experience as encountered at "the six sense gates": seeing, hearing, touching, tasting, smelling, and, from this perspective, thinking.

Reflecting for a moment, it becomes apparent that *all* experience has to come through these sense gates; without them, we cannot know the world. Observing experience at the sense gates shifts the focus of attention from *outside* us to *inside* us, from blame to the capacity to take responsibility for our own thoughts and feelings and the effect they have on others as well as ourselves.

Mindfulness Meditation, sometimes called Insight Meditation, is the form I use in my work. It's the oldest form of Buddhist meditation. Having emerged in India, it is currently practiced primarily in Southeast Asia, including Myanmar, Thailand, and Sri Lanka. When compared to Zen or Tibetan meditation, Mindfulness Meditation is the simplest, the least bound by the formality of ritual. Remarkably, it's also a close fit with our postmodern way of thinking in which reality becomes multifaceted, the self is composed of many and diverse parts, and knowledge shifts across time and context.

As the practice is described by my teacher, Shinzen Young, *mindfulness* is at the core. The word doesn't carry its ordinary meaning, which is to be vigilant about one's behavior, but instead refers to the process of bringing clarity and precision to awareness. The more complete instruction is to practice *mindfulness with equanimity*. Here, the definition of *equanimity* doesn't mean being passive or sitting on some imaginary mountaintop disengaged from the world. Instead, the word suggests the curious, matter-of-fact stance of a participant-observer. To maintain equanimity with your imagination, for instance, is to be both *in* a fantasy and *out* of it at the same time, an actor and an observer—not lost in the experience but, instead, watching it.

Shinzen briefly sums up the entire Mindfulness Meditation this way: *Bringing mindfulness and equanimity to ordinary experience leads to insight.* The word *insight* has at least two distinct meanings. As used in psychotherapy, it implies a surge of understanding into the personality. Uncovering shame, for instance, can come with the insight that it is rooted in early trauma rather than in a personal failing. As used in meditation, however, insight suggests an awareness of the larger whole; for example, one might get a glimpse into the *is-ness* of everything. From this perspective, there is no good or bad, no right or wrong. God makes room for the sinner and the saint.

The meditative tool for probing experience allows us to watch how thoughts arise and then fade, how powerful emotions such as anger or fear emerge and then subside. In this way we learn about the impermanence of experience. At one and the same moment we have a sense of the ever shifting, ephemeral nature of life and a more vibrant, deeper knowledge of it.[2]

MINDFULNESS PSYCHOTHERAPY

Over the past decade my work has slowly become a combination of psychotherapy and mindfulness meditation. I call it *Mindfulness Psychotherapy*, and I'm convinced that, for the Westerner, meeting the challenge that trouble brings by using both methods is more powerful than using either one alone. They fit together in many ways: both call for greater awareness, and through it, a conscious, increasingly precise study of the self; psychotherapy to enhance the self, meditation to let it go. Both offer the possibility of creating oneself anew.

There are several steps to the Mindfulness Psychotherapy practice. Each opens the door to a range of psychological and meditative awareness practices. No component stands alone, nor do the steps come in any particular order. Instead, they circle around each other in support of the total effort. Used collectively, they become a path toward wholeness. Here's a brief summary.

Naming Trouble

The act of giving experience a name is much like cleaving the waters of a deep and muddy river. What was a mystery suddenly becomes transparently clear. For example, if you're living with a vague sense of dis-ease and somehow become aware that your marriage is floundering, you're likely to be less confused, more focused.[3] Naming gives you the opportunity to think psychologically about when the problem began, who else is involved, how it patterns behavior, and what effects it has on other parts of your life. You can read about it, talk to friends, or join a support group. Our culture provides many opportunities for this exploration.

Naming the Emotions that Accompany Trouble

The truth is, trouble exists in the world. Even an illness or an addiction is, to some degree, external to the self. On the other hand, emotions exist inside us, in the feeling core of the body. The despair that can arise in a failing marriage or the fear that comes with a serious illness are deeply felt, internal responses to trouble. Because they go so deep, they can be nebulous and hard to distinguish. Naming these emotions, even if it is painful, produces a more authentic, genuine response to life. In the act of naming an emotion, what was a vague sense of disquiet that led nowhere, or a surge of anger that was instantly transformed into destructive behavior, becomes a pathway toward greater self-awareness. There are many ways of increasing your awareness of emotions. As you will see, Mindfulness Psychotherapy makes use of the relationship between the therapist and the client, using the meditative lens to focus on feelings in the body.

Cultivating Complete Acceptance

It's possible to name a problem but still continue to resist it—perhaps by drinking too much or by blaming others. Completely accepting the reality or the *is-ness* of an unhappy marriage, for example, means you know fully, deeply, that it exists. And completely accepting the is-ness of the anger you feel toward a partner means you sense the depth of the emotion. This acceptance doesn't necessarily imply expressing the anger or leaving the marriage. Nor does it imply suffering in silence.

Developing Equanimity

The word *equanimity* means that the emotions are in balance. This state of being can be seen in the matter-of-factness, the patience, and the capacity to suspend judgment that the scientist manifests when doing an experiment. In everyday life, equanimity gives us the freedom to know experience as it is—not as it's supposed to be. This same matter-of-factness allows us to accept the *reality* or the *is-ness* of trouble and the emotions that accompany it. As such, it goes a long way toward diminishing the suffering that comes with trouble. Equanimity is a skill that can be learned. We will focus on developing it in every one of these components that make up Mindfulness Psychotherapy.

Exploring the Mind/Body Process through Awareness

This meditative process begins as you hold trouble (perhaps a failing marriage) in your own two hands, look deeply inside yourself, and use your awareness to question what is going on. The first set of questions has to do with body sensations. What exactly is your body telling you about living in this marriage? For instance: *Are my muscles tight enough to be a suit of armor? Are there flutters in my abdomen? Do I feel like crying?*

Don't try to change those body sensations. Instead, *just feel*.

A second set of questions has to do with the mind. Once again, hold the marriage in your two hands and ask questions such as *Am I blaming my partner? Am I blaming myself? Is it hard to think about my marriage? Do I prefer to think about work or daydream about a vacation? Do I, instead, turn on the TV?*

Don't try to stop the mind. Instead, *just listen.*

Finally, hold the marriage in your two hands and observe the way you *see* it in night dreams, in daydreams, or, more generally, in your imagination. *Do these images reflect your sadness? Are they angry? Are they frightening?*

Don't try to do anything with the images. Instead, *just watch.*

As you will see, awareness leads to exquisitely clear observations of the mind/body process. With practice, and as your equanimity increases, the insights that heal are more likely to emerge.

Forming an Observing Self

Over time, you can develop the capacity observe the self during every-day life. While waiting for a bus or cooking a meal, you can listen to how you think, feel body sensations as they arise, and watch your dreams and fantasies. As awareness increases, this *observing self* grows increasingly knowledgeable and wise. What you will learn is that healing takes place repeatedly in different ways and at many moments as you move through the years.

Practicing Compassion

This path teaches that healing requires compassion—for yourself and for others. As you explore your own trouble and the emotions that accompany it, you're likely to realize that you're not too different from everyone else; each of us has our own particular form of trouble, along with our own particular form of suffering. Insight into the poignancy of the human condition leads to the development of compassion. We can help this natural process by nurturing the seeds of generosity and loving kindness that lie within us all. Practically speaking, this suggests the importance of self care, which includes eating healthy food, sleeping well, and getting sufficient exercise. It means congratulating yourself when you succeed at catching a glimpse of the mind/body process or find a degree of equanimity. And it advises affirming yourself if you feel compassion for yourself or anyone else on this troubled earth.

As you will see when you read the stories in this book, Mindfulness Psychotherapy can lead to a radical shift in one's relationship to life. The quest, which often begins as an attempt to get free from trouble, becomes a more expansive search for wholeness. When the doors of perception are unlocked, compassion enters. This is the love that embraces the lame and the whole, the disfigured and the beautiful. It's the love that leads toward peace.

THE DESIGN OF THE BOOK

Each chapter begins with a story—a woman's story, told in her own voice—which is followed by some thoughts about the journey both the woman and I took during the course of her therapy. In the first story, for instance, Tanya's capacity to manage terrible loss increased dramatically when she learned to live in the stillness that came with her suffering. For me, the challenge was holding the space for Tanya to grieve deeply. That wasn't easy, because I feared she would lose heart and move into a deep depression. Staying with her as she grieved demanded that I place my trust in the power of the healing relationship.

In another story, Kate's capacity to leave her abusive husband was made possible by an insight into the anger she carried around as a knot in her body. As she explored this reaction to her trouble, she learned an important truth: The body holds a certain wisdom that is grounding even as we go through great turmoil. And I discovered how to be with her even as she felt the rage that almost killed her.

In still another story, Nancy faced mental illness and almost died as a result. Ultimately she came to believe in herself and so emerged as a healer. Manifesting this archetype, she helped many women seek wholeness. The challenge for me was to remain grounded in the difference between mental illness and a spiritual awareness of that which others cannot see or hear.

These women are not very different from the rest of us. The troubles they faced are archetypal; in one way or another, we all struggle with them, whether in the form of the loss of a loved one, serious illness, or problems at work. And all these troubles come with difficult emotions. As you will see, the women learned how to use Mindfulness Meditation to heal them.

Each chapter ends with an opportunity for you, the reader, to have a direct experience of Mindfulness Meditation. The nine meditations in this book are designed to introduce you to the basics of a mindfulness practice and to teach you a way to heal emotions from troubles of your own. Many begin with an exercise that can help you settle in and also increase your capacity to concentrate. The meditations are progressively more challenging. You must decide how best to work with them. I'd suggest that if you're a beginner, you do each meditation as you read the book. After you have a sense of their progression, you can return to those that speak to you. However, if a particular meditation doesn't hold your attention, or if it's particularly disturbing, let it go. Perhaps you'll be ready to try it again after you've strengthened your meditative muscle.

After all, there's time. Meditation is a lifelong practice that is ever deepening and never finished.

I am deeply indebted to Shinzen Young for the clarity and precision with which he teaches Mindfulness Meditation. The meditations in *Emotional Healing through Mindfulness Meditation* are based on those he teaches.[4]

Learning meditation takes strong motivation, good instruction, and regular practice. Combining it with some form of psychotherapy, you can discover a deep-seated openness and acceptance of life. As you let go of the limiting conditions of the past, consciousness becomes purified and your personality begins to flow, like a wheel that has been well oiled.

Please remember that meditation is not easy. It is not a quick fix. If you practice for a half hour each day over several weeks, however, you can begin to experience the centeredness it offers. If you would like to hear, rather than read, the instructions, the compact disc included with this book offers the the meditations from chapters 1, 2, 3, and 5. You may choose to listen to the CD rather than reading the meditation instructions at the end of these chapters.

Mindfulness Psychotherapy is but one eddy in a powerful current moving through the helping professions at this time, a converging of the scientific and spiritual streams. If this surge of interest in the spiritual isn't engulfed by the more powerful materialist forces in our culture, the helping professions may very well teach us how to temper the individualism that results in loneliness with the holism that brings love and compassion. *Emotional Healing through Mindfulness Meditation* is an effort to understand how we can swim within this current, in the process bringing peace wherever it takes us in this world.[5]

One

How Tanya Found Her Song

There should have been some warning, some way of preparing for what was about to happen when I climbed out of bed that day, but there wasn't, so I simply stared out the window at the skeleton of a new building going up across the street. Rob, my lover of about two years, slept quietly behind me. Even the thought of him made me feel irritated; he was a medical machine, no heart. But we were planning to get married. Everybody thought it was time for me to settle down.

It had been an awful night. We had tried to make love, even though neither of us was very interested, so it was flat, dry. Of course we didn't talk about it; we rarely talked about anything. Yet we looked like a successful couple. Here I was, just on the edge of thirty, the music student with a great contralto voice who would someday be an opera star but who temporarily worked as a waitress. Meanwhile Rob, the newly graduated dermatologist, was a good doctor and on his way to making a lot of money.

As the sun rose, the hard hats began scampering over the girders. The one who wore a red neckerchief attracted me because he moved with such abandon even though burdened by heavy tools. I wasn't able to watch him for long because Rob woke up and began to get ready for work, so I withdrew to the kitchen. He appeared a half hour later dressed in his customary sport jacket and tie, and without so much as a nod of recognition, he poured himself a cup of coffee and left. The muscles in my neck loosened as he walked out the door.

Returning to the window, I caught another glimpse of the man in the red neckerchief and imagined I was up there with him, straddling a girder, legs dangling in space, hard hat securely on. Inspired, I put on the most beautiful dress in my closet and studied myself in the mirror. I must admit to liking the way the tight bodice enhanced the swelling of my breasts and the folds of sky blue silk exposed my sandaled feet. Placing a wide-brimmed straw hat on top of my long, dark brown hair, I blew a kiss toward the mirror and left the apartment.

I hope you won't judge me reckless, but the truth is, I walked ever so slowly in front of that construction site and relished the whistles and catcalls showering down upon me. I liked breaking the rules of proper behavior my mother had insisted on. It was my father who was the earthy one. I understood myself enough to know that I was caught between the two; I spent years dressing for my mother but behaving like my father. Walking down the street by the construction site on that day, I liked the attention I got, though I thought I shouldn't.

Looking up, I saw the man in the red neckerchief. He was watching me, so I waved up at him whimsically and then walked directly over to a local diner for breakfast. Sure enough, by the time I was seated, he arrived. That wasn't really surprising—I knew I could attract men. His name was Chuck, and he came on with that Marlboro Man kind of energy. I allowed a small smile to play over my lips. By the time breakfast was over we had a date to see each other the next night.

Much to my surprise, this game of mine became serious—and at a speed that left us breathless. True, when we kissed I felt guilty about being disloyal to Rob. And when I daydreamed about Chuck, my mother's disapproval boomed in my head. But every time I looked into his bottomless brown eyes or caught his muscles rippling underneath his shirt, I surrendered.

"Let's go for a spin on the motorcycle," he said one day. Of course I said yes. I knew it would be a blast. Careening around curves, we went at a speed that deserved to be illegal but felt like pure freedom. We both liked the special thrill we got by taking the risk of being caught. So we stole kisses on busy city streets and made love in the shadows of buildings late at night.

Neither of us was satisfied with the other parts of our lives. Chuck had broken up with his long-term lover, Sarah, two years before but still felt guilty about it and burdened by her constant demands. I desperately wanted to leave the music school I'd been going to for years; operatic singing was my mother's dream, not mine. Besides, Chuck and I hated city life; it was the natural world we wanted, a place where we could be ourselves.

Meanwhile, my relationship with Rob fell apart. Not that he fought for me; that wasn't his style. He didn't even ask where I spent my nights now that I wasn't sleeping at home. My family, however, was furious.

"Why can't you be satisfied with Rob?" my twin sister, Dawn, asked more than once. "Don't you know you're throwing your life away by hooking up with Chuck?"

Even my father disapproved. "What's the matter with you? Don't you know there's a difference between playing around and real life? Play with Chuck all you want, but marry Rob."

My mother stopped talking to me.

"Let's go to Canada," Chuck suggested soon after the day I moved into my own apartment. "This is our chance to make a new life. With my skills, I can get a job anywhere. And between us we have enough to put a down payment on a house somewhere in the mountains."

It was a great idea. We imagined ourselves horseback riding out in the wilderness. We thought about buying some chickens and a goat or two. And I always wanted to grow my own vegetables. Besides, I wouldn't have to set foot in that music school ever again.

Chuck wrote to a friend who was a construction worker in Vancouver, asking if he knew of any jobs in his part of the country. "Yes," came the answer booming through the mail. "Come on out! The pay is good." We decided to move on the one-year anniversary of our first meeting, which gave us four months to pack up and say good-bye.

My family was upset about the move and complained loudly. But

Sarah, Chuck's former lover, was devastated. It meant he would never return to her. I could hear her scream hysterically when they tried to talk on the phone. "You can't do this to me," she cried. "You promised to move back home this summer. Please, I need you. Your mother needs you. Don't do it."

As the moving date approached, we gave notice at our jobs, sold whatever furniture we had, and bought a camper with a rack on the back for Chuck's motorcycle. I packed up my city clothes and stored them in my sister's attic. Friends gave us a great farewell party. Life couldn't have been better.

And then, two days before we were to leave, Sarah called in the middle of the night to say that her mother had just had a heart attack and was at death's door. She pleaded with Chuck to visit once more before her mother died.

"Please don't go," I cried. "That woman will do anything to get you back, even say that her mother's deathly ill."

"Don't worry," Chuck insisted. "Remember, Sarah doesn't mean anything to me anymore. It's you I love. We're going to spend the rest of our lives together. Anyway, I owe it to Sarah's mother to say good-bye before she dies. No matter what I think about Sarah, her mother was always good to me. Besides, my friend Dave just came back into town, so I'll be able to see him before we leave. I'll drive up early this afternoon and be back tomorrow morning."

Still, I pleaded with him to stay away from Sarah. "I don't trust her. Promise me you won't go over to her house or ask for anything you left behind, not even the guitar."

"I promise, I promise," he said repeatedly as he prepared to leave, but I knew he didn't mean it. When Chuck had the impulse to do something, he did it. He was being drawn to Sarah like a moth to a flame.

I was still asleep very early the next morning when the phone rang. It was Dave. There were tears in his voice: "I hate to be the one who has to tell you this, but somebody has to. Please forgive me. Don't blame me."

Choking on his words, he finally blurted out his awful message: "Tanya, Chuck's *dead*. Sarah *killed* him."

"What? What did you say?" I thought I hadn't heard right.

"He went to visit Sarah last night, I suppose to say good-bye before the two of you left. And Tanya, I can't believe it's true, but Sarah *shot* him. She actually *shot him in the chest*. He died on the spot."

Having begun to talk, this poor man couldn't stop. "I don't know what to say. It's awful. Just horrible. What should I do? Should I come down to get you? Are you all right? What do you want me to do?"

Feeling numb, I mumbled a few words of good-bye and called my sister. A couple of hours later Dawn and I were driving upstate, still hoping against all hope that it was a bad dream. But when we saw Chuck's body at the local morgue, we knew it wasn't. The police captain told us Sarah had confessed. It seems she asked Chuck to make love one more time, and when he refused, she slipped the gun out from underneath a pillow on the couch and shot him. Apparently they had been drinking a lot; there was an empty bottle of Scotch on the coffee table.

Not much else Sarah said made any sense, the officer reported. She was in jail now, but her lawyer was insisting she be transferred to a hospital for an evaluation of her mental status.

Too soon, the funeral was over. Dawn and I came home to grieve in my nearly empty apartment. There was nothing to do but grieve. For days on end we sat half-reclining at either end of a shabby tweed couch, legs tucked underneath and heads resting against some bedraggled old pillows. I couldn't stop crying.

I remember bits and pieces of that time with great clarity; the images stand out against a very dark background. I know we went over the story of his death thousands of times, trying hard to figure it out, and wishing we could somehow make the ending come out differently.

And then there was the time Dawn asked, "Why did he fall for Sarah's story to begin with?"

"I guess he still wanted Sarah to forgive him. But if he knew he didn't want to have sex with her, why did he go back to her apartment?"

"Maybe he was caught by the offer of a drink," Dawn responded. "The only good times those two ever had were when they drank."

"But why would she *kill* him?" I cried, as my body began to shake with a rage I didn't know I had. "I wish she was here so I could pound on her, beat her, *kill* her."

I was shocked at the strength of my anger and tried to control myself. "Oh God, why did Chuck let her back into his life? I knew she was crazy. Why didn't I *demand* that he stay home with me? I sensed the evil inside her but I didn't do anything about it! Why didn't I listen to my intuition?"

And then my pulse quickened again and I felt that rage swelling in every pore of my body. I saw images of myself thrusting a knife into Sarah's heart thousands of times, heard her cry for mercy, and my heart was glad. She was evil and deserved to die. "I *will* kill her, I'll find her and *kill* her. That's what I'll do. I'll *kill* her. *I will!* Chuck would want me to do it, I know he would."

In a flood of tears, my rage collapsed. "I didn't protect the man I loved. Dear lord, I wish I had the will to kill her. I wish I did."

As you might imagine, this really frightened Dawn. She didn't know what to do with me, except to try to get me to see a therapist. For days after, she talked about this. She even got the telephone number of someone her friend had seen.

"What can a therapist do?" I argued. "No one can bring him back. Besides, you know I'm a private person. I don't want to wash my dirty laundry in someone's office."

So I never made an appointment, even though the rage came back many times. I planned Sarah's death while I was awake and committed murder in my nightmares. Then, as abruptly as it came, the rage went, leaving me feeling both relieved and hopeless. "That woman killed the man I love, and no one is going to do anything about it. I bet she'll claim insanity and be free in no time at all."

We couldn't have known then that several months later my sister and I would sit in the courtroom and listen while Sarah was found not guilty by reason of insanity and remanded to a state institution for the criminally insane. Two years later, she was free.

At first glance you wouldn't guess Dawn and I were sisters, let alone that she was only four minutes older. People said I was good-looking in a sophisticated sort of way, especially when I pulled my dark hair back in a French knot and dressed in simple black. Dawn had the same high forehead and clear blue eyes, but she was twenty pounds over-weight and dressed like the homemaker and mother of two that she was.

I don't know what I would have done without her; she watched me cry and rage with remarkable patience, and in between, she found ways to make me laugh. "Remember the frilly aqua dress Mom made you for our high school graduation party? And how you stomped around and raved about not wearing it *anywhere,* especially to your graduation party? You actually showed up in dirty old jeans."

"I was always in trouble. Remember the guys I picked to go out with during high school, and the trouble I got into? The only way I can explain it is that our family needed a rebel and Dad had resigned from the role."

"You're just like Dad," Dawn added, "a blue-collar soul caught in stockings and heels. Remember how he complained about the suit he had to wear on Sundays, or when he had to take his shoes off before coming into the house? He hated the rules Mom imposed on us. So did you.

"Let me tell you a secret," she continued in a quiet voice. "I was always jealous of you. Even now I am. You have the looks and that beautiful voice. And I'm just a housewife stuck in the suburbs. It was always that way. I was the good little girl, doing just what Mama said, and you were the rebel."

"Wait a minute, you've got it wrong," I replied, surprised. "I was the one who envied you! Give me half a chance and I did something wrong. I either spilled milk all over Mom's kitchen floor or had holes in my jeans. Dad never complained, but Mom made up for it by being all over both of us. We were the outcasts: Dad, the factory worker who never made enough money, and Tanya, the twin who never learned manners. Meanwhile, everything you did was great. I could never set a table like you did. And Mom loved you for it."

"Oh, come on," my sister groaned, lifting her eyebrows in disbelief. "I fit in just like the needlepoint of *God Bless Our Home* that hung on the kitchen wall. No one ever saw me."

During one particularly dreary night I became terribly aware of the bare white walls and the bleakness of the apartment. The place had an eerie, empty feel about it, as if it were a tomb waiting for a body. *Maybe it should be mine,* said a voice inside, a just punishment for not protecting Chuck.

In that uncanny way of hers, Dawn knew I was heading for dangerous territory. She roused herself, held my head against her chest, and said, "Try not to torture yourself, my little sister. Chuck's death wasn't your fault. You couldn't have stopped him from going back to Sarah and her mother if you tied him up. He was always a guy who did what he wanted. He took risks, even on the job. Remember the time he did a handstand for you on a steel girder a hundred feet above the ground?"

Ready to end the conversation, she stretched, peeled herself loose from the couch, and gave me a great hug. "We're so lucky to have each other," she whispered in my ear. "And now, my dear, the clock says three A.M. It's time for me to go to bed."

A familiar surge of panic tore though me; I was frightened of what my mind would conjure up without my sister next to me. "Don't go to sleep yet," I begged. "Don't leave me alone."

But she insisted. "Come on, enough is enough. Grab hold of yourself. You're beautiful and you're talented. That voice of yours will carry you through."

There was nothing to do but make the best of it, so clothes and all, I climbed into bed and closed my eyes. Dozing off, I heard the sounds of the city, the wind, police sirens, the noise of traffic rising and falling as if I were in the middle of an ocean. In the dream that came, I *was* in the ocean, in a small rowboat that seemed destined to be swamped by the next big wave. My stomach dropped with each fall. Feeling desperate, I used every bit of strength to try to reach the shore, but I didn't quite know where that was.

Rob appeared at the other end of the boat. He looked like death warmed over. Even in my dream I realized he always looked like that. How could I ever have hooked up with him? He was such a wimp.

"Tanya," he called out. "Help me! You know I can't swim. I'm afraid of drowning. Save me."

"Sit down, you idiot," I yelled back. "Sit down and row." It was a waste of breath. He kept trying to reach me. The boat was just about to tip and then, out of the corner of my eye, I saw Chuck! He was there—

really there! He was in his work clothes, hard hat and all, exactly the way he was dressed when I met him a year ago. "Don't worry baby, I'm here to help," he said. "I'm not going to let you go under. I love you too much."

"Oh Chuck, I'm so glad to see you," I screamed above the roar of the ocean. "Help me, please help me. I can't do it alone."

Turning toward the horizon, I saw a monstrous wave rolling toward us. "Look, look," I shouted.

"Point the bow into the wave and pull hard on the oars," he ordered calmly, even as we sank into the deep depression that came before the swell. "Meet it head on, honey. Head on. And don't be afraid."

Much to my relief, the boat made it over the swell.

"I'll always be here when you need me," Chuck said. "I'll give you the strength you need."

Next thing I knew, the boat and the waves were gone and I heard myself calling out, "Chuck, don't leave, don't leave." When I opened my eyes, Dawn was at my side, wiping my brow and trying to comfort me. "Shh, honey, shh. Everything is going to be all right. I'm here now."

"I *saw* him," I sobbed. "I *saw* him. But was it really Chuck? Or was it a dream? I don't know. I don't know. Am I going crazy? I could have sworn he was alive. He was so real."

There was nothing to do but cry. And that, too, finally ended. Exhausted, hoping my words would prove to be true, I said, "No more crying. No more thinking. I can't do it anymore. There's nothing more to say or feel or do. I'm tired."

Finally the time came when Dawn had to go back home. Her husband was weary of all the attention she was giving me and annoyed by her absence. And the children needed her. It was time; I had to find my own way. So I went back to work as a waitress, sold the camper and the motorcycle, bought new furniture for the apartment, and found a therapist. Barbara was her name.

Still, I felt as if I were living a nightmare. I wasn't much interested in anything or anyone. Why even try? Nothing I did, no relationship, would last for long. I even managed to alienate my friends. It was as though I put a sign on my door saying, *Stay Away!*

But I still had Chuck. His clothes hung in my closet; his leather jacket was draped over the arm of the couch. I liked to nuzzle into his clothes because the scent reminded me of him. Often I heard his voice calling me, and looking around I thought I even saw him. Sometimes in the middle of the night I felt him lying next to me, and turning over to snuggle, I'd realized what I felt was a phantom body, a ghost. And when images of making love arose in my mind, nothing could ease the ache.

I was surprised that Barbara didn't think I was crazy. She said I was suffering from a mind that was unable to accept the reality of Chuck's death, and that I would grieve until the mind could do it. I didn't know quite what she meant, but I did get that she thought grieving was what I had to do. So I cried and rambled through my history. She listened and often gave me a hug. Each time I left her office I felt better.

There came a time of some relief. Chuck faded enough for me to put on my fine clothes and walk past some construction sites. I went out on a number of dates but never did find another Chuck. I even wrote to a prisoner in a local jail, thinking that, because we were both outsiders, I'd be able to talk to him. But that didn't work either. And then grief grabbed hold of me again. This time, it really frightened me. Would it ever end? But my therapist kept encouraging me to ride it out; she assured me that my mind would eventually settle in and I would learn something important.

And so, wave after wave of my mournful life broke upon me, soaking, scrubbing, denying me even a dream of happiness. That became a fantasy only normal people could indulge in. Mine was a different route. But what that route was still escaped me. I had no plan, no wish for the future. I even stopped worrying about it. And slowly, over the months, I felt a strange kind of peace: the peace that comes with not caring about anything more than the next step. It was okay. In fact, I kind of liked the feeling. Besides, I didn't feel alone—if the night got too murky or I were in real trouble, I knew Chuck would always be there. In the flick of an eye I could catch sight of him or hear his voice. He was keeping me alive. And my therapist didn't think I was crazy. She even said I was doing well!

Then, on one rather mundane evening after work, I put on the radio and caught the music of Billie Holiday. The sound was riveting. This was singing I understood! Something I instinctively knew how to do. Why hadn't I ever paid attention to the blues before? It isn't that I had never listened to Billie Holiday sing. I had, many times.

I felt Chuck encouraging me to sing along with her on the radio. Long after the music stopped, he continued singing, urging me on. I would hear him singing the blues as I showered or catch a few lines while sitting in a bus. I finally got the message.

So I decided to learn more about the blues. I went to live performances, got myself a singing coach, and practiced. I even found an accompanist, and together we honed an act. The blues became my way out of grieving. I didn't know where it would take me, but that didn't matter. I had a new life.

People liked my singing. I think they were captivated by the intensity they could feel behind the words. They probably also sensed I was singing to someone who wasn't there, and they were right. That someone was Chuck. I cried to him, laughed with him, grieved for him, all in front of an audience. In response, Chuck whispered soft words of support. I was baring my love in public, and it gave many of the souls in front of me the freedom to do the same, in private.

After years had passed and my music had grown strong, the pain of Chuck's death actually began to fade. Even his visits became less frequent. And I didn't feel lonely anymore. Strangely enough, neither did I want another man. Singing had become my life, as important as breathing. I was living a miracle.

I began to write my own music. Getting up early in the morning, I would try out a new tune. Going to work, snatches of songs would bubble up. When I climbed into bed at night, arrangements swirled through my mind. To my amazement, the music was joyful as well as melancholy. It told of loss and survival, of death and rebirth.

Without any agent or public relations effort, almost without my awareness, more and more people came to hear me sing. The room was often full. My childhood dream had come true; I was a star! What really made life sweet, though, were those times when I reached out to someone in the audience and sensed a kindred soul.

I found my song, and it bonded me with a world of others.

> *Live as if you liked yourself, and it may happen:*
> *reach out, keep reaching out, keep bringing in.*
> *This is how we are going to live for a long time, not always,*
> *for every gardener knows that after the digging, after the planting,*
> *after the long season of tending and growth, the harvest comes.*
>
> —MARGE PIERCY

FINDING THE STILLNESS

I'll never forget the first time I met Tanya. She seemed so forlorn that I couldn't help but fear she would kill herself. As she told her story, however, my fear subsided. Tanya was searching for something in all her grieving, and I sensed that the search itself would keep her alive.

Women throughout the ages have grieved as intensely as Tanya did, sometimes even more so. They have wailed and howled, torn their clothes and pulled out their hair—all to make peace with death. However, this is not how we grieve in our time. We are more contained. So contained that we often lose the opportunity to find our way through such terrible loss. As a people, whenever trouble arises we tend to short-circuit our feelings and move quickly toward solutions that offer immediate comfort. Many of us might think that a more acceptable response to Tanya's terrible loss would be for her to take some medication, be sad for a couple of months, and then go out and buy herself a brand new red convertible.

I often wonder what it is that makes us think that we can use *things* to erase trouble from our lives, that we can take a pill or buy a new car and all will be well. What a powerful spell our culture casts to convince so many of us that material comfort is the answer to human suffering. It doesn't make sense! How can a new car or a diamond ring heal the terrible loneliness that comes with the loss of a loved one? How can alcohol or a pill be anything more than a temporary answer to abuse?

This belief in comfort doesn't reflect the truth that trouble is part of life and can't be wished away. It also obscures the truth that trouble exists not only in the outside world but also inside, in emotions that persist even after we get the new car or the diamond ring. Most important, this belief in comfort obscures the truth that trouble contains the germ of its own resolution as well as the potential for personal transformation.

Tanya's story is important because she did, indeed, experience a transformation *in the very process of grieving her loss.* The story of her healing began as she and I created what has been called by Donald Winnicott a *holding environment,* a safe place to pursue grieving and the search that is embedded within it. It is a place designed to be fully accepting, respectful, and dependable.[1] In this context, Tanya found the courage to grieve for as long as she needed, and she found the determination, the stick-to-it-ness, that leads to healing. It happened through Mindfulness Psychotherapy.

Naming the trouble was our first challenge. It wasn't as easy for Tanya as one might think, because naming and accepting the *is-ness* of Chuck's death were wrapped together inside her mind. From the very beginning, on the day he died, she had trouble acknowledging his death, partly because it was sudden, but also because it destroyed the future they had created. Certainly going through the steps of identifying the body, speaking to the police, and going to the funeral helped make it real, but the words *Chuck is dead* still didn't feel right inside. Even months after he died, she kept trying to keep him alive, because she needed him. Indeed, he helped her learn how to sing the blues—but that came later, after she was more able to let him go.

Naming the emotions that come with the trouble turned out to be a fruitful therapeutic endeavor. Tanya was curious about her emotions. They interested her. She was aware, for instance, that she felt nothing right after Chuck's death. It worried her. She even wondered if this absence of feeling meant she didn't love him. But soon enough the horror of his death had seeped in. And that was followed by a rage that made her want to kill. And under it all was a deep despair. It took great courage not to run from such emotions. And they didn't go away even after many months of grieving! Secretly, she thought she might be going crazy. That, indeed, is what brought her into therapy.

The extremes of human experience trigger extreme emotional reactions. Having a loved one murdered, for instance, can induce horror and rage. It can even produce the "extrasensory" perception that the murdered person is still alive. This is the mind desperately—and very creatively—trying to make sense of the experience. The problem is that we often become frightened of the very grieving we need to do and believe, instead, that we're going crazy. Then it's most likely we'll force the mind back to commonplace thinking and so lose the opportunity to work our way through our trouble.

Fortunately, Tanya didn't do that. Actually, she was one of those people who can't stop grieving, even if they want to. She had to find her way through, and therapy offered the opportunity. During one therapy session, when she heard Chuck talking to her and thought she was going crazy, I held her closely in my gaze, slowed down my speech, and reassured her that this was part of the grieving process. As her breathing slowed, I asked her to listen to Chuck's voice and be aware of the feeling it triggered. So she watched the feeling of panic rise and fall like a great wave inside her. To her surprise, the panic didn't overwhelm her; in fact, it slowly dissipated.

This was the kind of work we did together many times, not only with panic, but also with rage, horror, and despair. Slowly these emotions lost their charge. Indeed, by watching her fear of going crazy over time, it eventually disappeared. And Chuck's voice became more comfortable to live with, not as a sign of mental illness but as part of the grieving process.

Stillness was the first great gift of all this effort to heal Tanya's emotions. It came with the slowing down of time that allowed her to sense the beating of her heart and the ebb and flow of her breath. Her mind itself quieted down—and yet it was focused. There was no fear, no guilt, just deep sadness, and then a few precious moments of peace. Once she told me she felt cradled in those moments, held in the silence. Chuck wasn't present, and yet she felt loved.

From that stillness came her second great gift—the blues. Singing was a conduit, a funnel through which she could give voice to her grief. People who would never have such a terrible experience of loss sensed her grief. Those who had had such experiences understood. Singing became her route back to everyday life. And when someone was able to hear her songs deeply, it filled her with great joy. That joy was an affirmation of her path.

On Healing

As you read the following chapters, you will see that every one of the women engaged in the practice of Mindfulness Psychotherapy. Although the seven components of the process didn't come in any particular order, each woman *named her trouble* and then *named the accompanying emotions*. Sometimes the naming was hard—especially if she had grown accustomed to living with confusion. Clarity hurt as the reality emerged. It was also difficult for those who had hidden emotions such as shame, guilt, fear, or despair for years on end. Each emotion stung painfully as it was finally felt.

Finding her way toward a *complete acceptance* of trouble, and the emotions that came with it, each woman understood that her emotions were sometimes causing more suffering than the trouble itself. Often, much to her surprise, a complete acceptance of the *is-ness* of emotions didn't drown her in a sea of feeling. Paradoxically, she actually began to feel bigger than her emotions, more free of them. And so her suffering was reduced.

For some, this was their first taste of *equanimity*—the balanced mind. They developed a greater capacity for being matter-of-fact and nonjudgmental. This gave them the freedom to explore the *mind/body process* that gave rise to suffering. Slowly, by learning how to use awareness as a tool, most of these women understood that, because suffering is grounded in the mind/body process, it can be diminished.

As time went on and exploration became part of everyday life, every woman, at least to some degree, developed an *observing self*. In this way, the practice began to transform daily experiences. New people, new talent, new opportunities arose.

Finally, the search for *compassion* took its place in the women's healing. They grew to recognize the seeds of it in themselves. And they nurtured those seeds. Healing couldn't have taken place without compassion for themselves and others.

A few went further on the path to wholeness and used meditation to develop a *spiritual life*. Trouble might have been the reason they began, but they continued in order to know the buoyancy, the humility, and the uncanny insight that come with states of stillness. After long practice, they learned how to experience life holistically and so touch the larger whole or feel held in the hands of God. At first this seemed extraordinary. But after much effort, when they finally did catch a glimpse of that state in themselves, it actually turned out to be rather ordinary, something that just was. The same can be said for the stars and the Milky Way. They are truly miraculous, and they just are.

On Meditation

The meditation at the end of this chapter is about finding stillness. Especially in a culture like ours, in which people are addicted to ever changing sensations and constant activity, stillness is a special gift. So addicted are we to busyness that we forget the experience of having nothing to do. We forget that this state can offer many riches: the sound of the wind, the touch of the air as it brushes our skin, the sight of a hawk soaring through the sky, the experience of being. And the meditative instruction is: Just be aware.

What does *just be aware* mean? It means being continuously mindful. For example, in a few moments I will ask you to make the body the object of your meditation—two arms, two legs, a torso, and a head. Doing this may make you more aware of the vibrancy, the aliveness of it. In this case, being aware means being continuously in touch with whatever sensations arise in the body. The challenge is to sustain that awareness matter-of-factly, with curiosity. Being matter-of-fact is a skill. It's the stance of the scientist while he or she watches the paths of subatomic particles in a cloud chamber or the eating habits of the great ape in the jungle. It takes curiosity, patience, and a calm mind.

Now, an interesting thing will probably happen as you try to be mindful of the body: thoughts will interrupt. Soon you will find yourself thinking about something that must be done, something you forgot to do, something you didn't do well. You might even create a fantasy, and before you know it you're on a beach in Hawaii. The mind keeps us busy. It cuts us off us from the experience of being. When this happens—and it will happen repeatedly—the meditative instruction is once again: Just be aware.

Don't try to ignore your inner voice, or stop it, or in anyway control it. Simply accept its presence. Here's the key: Make it background to your meditation. When you're focusing on the breath moving through the body, expect thoughts to come and go, and as soon as you recognize their presence, return to the focus of the meditation. This sounds easy. But it isn't. You will repeatedly get caught by the power of the next thought and so lose the focus on your body. Time will pass before you realize what's happening. That's okay. Simply return to the body.

Alternatively, feelings can arise. You might feel irritable, antsy, resentful, controlled. You are asking the mind/body process to slow down, to follow an instruction, and it resists. Again, the instruction is to return to the object of your meditation. Eventually you will be able to do so.

The goal of meditation isn't simply to concentrate on the body. We learn to stay with the body so we can understand what it has to teach. What is the nature of the body sensation that comes with fear? Is it clear or subtle? How does it change? How long does it last? What do we have to learn from it, or from any other experience of life? The purpose of meditation is to penetrate experience, to see things as they are. We don't avoid, run away from, or argue with a sensation or a feeling. We slow down and learn to live in stillness so that we can watch a thought or a sensation with curiosity, matter-of-factly, without trying to control it or change it. And then we see that it changes by itself. Over time, this practice can be applied to the rest of life.

Before we begin this first meditation, let's take a few moments to consider certain basics. For instance, holding the right posture is important. When you meditate, keep your spine straight and your ears in line with the shoulders. Relax those shoulders, tilt your head slightly forward, and tuck in your chin. Try not to tilt sideways, backward, or forward. Sit as if there were a string between the sky and the top of your head. Keep your hands on your thighs or in your lap, palms up in a cupped position, with the left cup in the right cup. This gives your posture strength. It's your body at its best, strong and relaxed, expressive of its own nature. The posture is symbolic. You don't mold yourself into the chair or shape yourself for others; instead, you exist as you are, hanging on your own spine. At first the posture may be hard to maintain, but eventually you will find it comfortable.[2]

It's traditional to sit cross-legged on a cushion; however, you can also hold the posture in a straight-backed chair by sitting slightly forward, perhaps with a pillow under your feet. You can even hold it standing up. Often it helps to change positions, especially when you're a beginner, so please feel free to shift while you're doing the meditations that follow. But do so slowly, and stay aware of the subtle changes in your body as you move.

Soon you will see that sitting isn't always easy. You might hear yourself think, *I'm uncomfortable; I'm getting hungry, I have to go to the bathroom, I'm annoyed with the constraints of the posture.* That the body craves so much attention is an important insight.

You might also hear yourself think, *I'm not doing it well. I'm not cut out for this. What's wrong with me?* Of course, it can go the other way: *I'm a natural-born meditator. I'm fantastic. Others will soon see how good I am.*

Both kinds of judgment present the same problem. They separate you from the experience. When you finally have moments that aren't filled with the constant haranguing of the *I,* you will actually have a sense of peace. And if, at the end of the following meditation, you don't think you've been able to keep the focus, remember that even just a few brief moments of stillness are important. They massage the spiritual substance of your being and deepen your sense of life as it is.

It's important to say that Mindfulness Meditation isn't a magic potion. Rather, it's a precise inquiry into the mind/body process—a method that, fortunately, has been laid out by generations upon generations of meditators who came before. Because of them, the path is more accessible.

The meditation that follows offers an experience of stillness. I'm grateful to my teacher, Shinzen, for teaching it to me. Please be aware that the experience of stillness shifts in quality and intensity as you become more experienced. Perhaps at this point in your practice you will be able to find the quiet and the relaxation that are often the first taste of this state of being. With years of practice you may be able to find a stillness that is both exquisitely quiet and deeply sustaining.

To begin, find a quiet space, choose a cushion or a chair with a straight back, and to the degree you can, protect yourself from external sound. And please have patience with yourself.

Try listening to this meditation by using the compact disc that comes with this book; hearing the guidance can make the meditation more alive. If you choose to follow the printed instructions, begin by reading the entire meditation first, noting how each paragraph contains new instructions. If you like, use the memory prompt in the summary at the end of the meditation.

Because this meditation is designed to calm the mind, I will ask you to repeat it before many of the other meditations in this book. For this reason, you might want to memorize it.

At appropriate times, I'll cue you to put down the book so you can take more time to soak in that particular experience. Place a timer by your side so you can measure the length of time you meditate by yourself. And if it helps you keep track of your progress, take some notes.

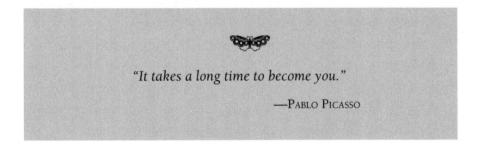

"It takes a long time to become you."

—Pablo Picasso

A Meditation on Finding the Stillness

Close your eyes and take a moment to let the body settle. Allow your shoulders to drop an inch or two.

Now make the object of your awareness the body . . . specifically the right side of the body . . . just the right side. Scan the length of it . . . the width of it . . . the breadth of it. Cover as much of it as possible. As best you can, be aware of the right side of the body.

Note the difference between the right side and the left side.

Then let go of the right side and make the object of your awareness the left side of the body . . . just the left side. Be aware of how it stretches out into space along its length and along its width. Sense its depth.

When you're ready, bring the two sides together, right and left, into one unified whole. Cover that whole volume of feeling space with awareness . . . experience it all . . . the length . . . the width . . . the depth of that body space. Sit with an awareness of the whole body.

❦

Let go of that, and make the object of awareness the front of the body . . . just the front. Soak its length with awareness. Soak its width with awareness.

Now bring your awareness to the back of the body . . . just the back. Soak that with awareness . . . both its length and its width.

Finally, bring the two together, front and back, into an entire whole. Feel how the whole body becomes more alive when it receives this attention.

❦

Let go of that, and make the object of awareness the upper half of the body, both back and front. Feel it as a volume that has a back and a front and a depth. Be aware. Two arms . . . half of the torso . . . a neck . . . a head.

Now, shift your awareness to the lower half of your body. Scan its length . . . its width . . . its depth. Half a torso . . . two legs . . . two feet . . . ten toes. Be aware.

Now include both the upper and the lower halves of the body in the same awareness. Feel the volume of feeling space . . . a head . . . two arms . . . two legs . . . and a torso. An integrated . . . fully functioning . . . whole. Sense the vibrancy of it.

Please put down the book at this point and use this meditation strategy by yourself. Set your timer for five minutes.

❦

After five minutes have passed, slowly open your eyes and sit quietly . . .
preserving the stillness even as you let everyday life in through your eyes.
Feel the slowness of your breathing, the relaxation of the body. These few
moments are important. They give you a glimpse of how it's possible to pre-
serve the stillness in the midst of everyday life.

❈

Take a moment to think of a trouble that you have, perhaps an unhappy
marriage or the illness of a child. In the stillness, name it. Try to accept the
is-ness of it, the reality that this trouble exists. And sit quietly for a while.

Then slowly stand up, once again feeling the stillness in your body. As
you go about the rest of your day, remember that stillness from time to time
. . . and be aware that you can return to it whenever you want.

May all beings know stillness.

Training for Awareness

1. Bring your awareness to the right side of the body and scan for
   sensations. Do the same for the left side. Do the same for the
   whole body.

   Repeat this sequence for the front half of the body, the back
   half, and the whole body.

   Repeat this sequence for the top half of the body, the bottom
   half, and the whole body.

2. Give a name to something that is troubling you. Accept the
   is-ness of it.

Two

Kate's Loving Addiction

The story I'm about to tell you began eight years ago on a sunny afternoon just before I found the letters. The memory stands out bright and clear, perhaps because everything became a dull gray soon afterward. I was waiting for Gary in our beautiful new bedroom, my interior designer's dream come true. Surrounded on three sides by windows that stretched from floor to ceiling, the room had an oval-shaped spa and antique English furniture. From the king-sized bed I could look through the windows and see a tall oak and an ancient elm spread their canopies over the expanse of lawn behind the house. Usually I loved to look out those windows, but that afternoon I was edgy and a little bored.

It's embarrassing to tell you that I spent a lot of time thinking about the good-looking guy who had worked out next to me in the gym that morning. However, when I heard Gary's car turn into the driveway, I got out of bed and examined myself in the mirror. My body was trim in its spandex polo shirt and tight jeans, but not quite trim enough. My stomach bulged a little, and I bemoaned the fact that my muscles weren't as tight as they used to be. The exercise routine I was doing with my personal trainer was making a difference, but it wasn't enough. I secretly believed the only thing that would really help was being ten years younger.

"Mmm, you smell good today," I murmured, greeting Gary in the hallway.

He said nothing but grabbed for my left breast. It made me cringe. Why was he so crude, such a boor? Trying to hide my distaste, I picked up his Ferragamo raincoat and hung it in the closet.

Meanwhile Gary admired his new haircut in the hall mirror. "I had some time this afternoon so I tried out the new men's salon next to the health club. Didn't they do a good job, Kate?" Noticing my nod wasn't particularly friendly, he quipped, "All for my sales career."

As I tried to move past him, he turned abruptly, wrapped his arms around my waist, and pulled me up against him sharply. I groaned inside. What did he think I was, a toy? This was far from the romantic scene I had been imagining while lying in bed. But there was no more time to think; his voice flat, Gary was suggesting we have a quickie before our eight-year-old son came home from his soccer game.

Glancing at my watch, I calculated we had thirty minutes until our son came home. This would really have to be quick. I had dinner to make. So, with a certain reluctance that Gary probably noticed, I said okay. He took that as an opportunity to touch a pimple on my face and grimace his disapproval. I felt awful about the pimple; it was so humiliating. I remember wishing I could get away to put on some more makeup, but at the time, I could no more have gotten away than fly to the moon.

I hope you understand that this is very hard for me to tell you. I've come a long distance since that afternoon, and if it happened now, I wouldn't let him be so mean to me. But that day I didn't feel as if I had any choice; all I could do was try to stay calm. Besides, I loved Gary.

"Strip for me, Kate," he half asked, half demanded, and without waiting for an answer, he quickly undressed and propped himself up on the bed to watch. "And don't make it boring. Throw yourself into it this time, like you used to years ago."

I did just as he asked.

Pulling the shirt over my head, I exposed my bare skin inch by inch and finally cupped my breasts as if to make an offering. I brushed my hair in repetitive arcs in front of the mirror so he could see my breasts bob and neck arch, all the while worrying whether this would work.

Gary didn't like my breasts. He said they were "droopy" and actually wanted me to get them tightened by a plastic surgeon.

"Oh, well," I thought to myself, "maybe I'll get around to it some-day."

I kicked off my shoes and peeled my jeans down over my hips, turning so he could get a good view. Seeing a flicker of excitement in his eyes, I realized I didn't have to worry; my performance was beginning to work. "Not bad," I thought, and I actually began to enjoy myself.

It was a well-rehearsed ritual, so we both knew what would happen next. Moving into bed, I stretched out next to him and moaned my readiness. Without any attempt at caressing, he lifted his heavy body on top of mine and entered in. I needed to shift positions to be more comfort-able, but this was dangerous—if I annoyed him, he might lose his erec-tion, and that would make him angry. Fortunately, I managed it without a problem. He moved harshly and came quickly. He didn't ask if I had. No matter; the sex was over and I could get out of bed. The chicken had to be fried.

Back in the kitchen, Gary kissed me on the neck, murmuring, "That was good." I responded with a long and slightly seductive "Yes," but actually I felt annoyed by the closeness of his body. So, without think-ing, I placed my hand on his chest and nudged, or as he felt it, shoved him away.

His good mood collapsed like a perforated balloon. Catching sight of a laundry basket overflowing with dirty clothes, he remembered he had only one pair of clean underwear left in his drawer that morning, and told me so. Scanning the kitchen counters, he added that the house was as messy as it was when he left for work. Tasting the chicken, he exploded. "This stuff tastes like cardboard! Your cooking is terrible! And you haven't even set the table. What exactly did you do all day?"

It was the beginning of a tirade I had heard many times before: "My mother wouldn't be seen dead serving a meal like this. I think you should take lessons from her. Maybe she's the one who can get through to you. I can't."

If I didn't calm him down, there was no telling what might happen, so I quickly apologized. "I'm sorry, Gary, I should have set the table, but

I didn't have the time. Please don't get angry at me. I'll try to do better next time."

The apology didn't help. "Every surface has your junk on it. Look around you, really *look*. I offer you a magnificent environment, pay for everything, even get someone to clean up after you, and all I get in return is a mess! No thanks, no gratitude, or for that matter, no peace. Just a mess."

Even in my fear, I was struck by the hurt in his voice. "What I want is a woman who's there for me. My mother did that for my father. Why can't you do that for me? When he came home at night there was good food, an elegantly prepared table, and a beautiful wife. But you, you don't know how to cook and you don't know how to dress. I can't figure it out. Are you out to destroy me, or are you just plain crazy?"

I stood very still, wishing I could disappear. It was all my fault. He needed something from me that I wasn't giving him. I couldn't cook and I couldn't clean. I was a failure. Once again I was a little girl being yelled at by my father.

"I'm sorry I'm so stupid. I'm sorry, I'm sorry," I said to him as I had said to my father after I had disappointed him. That was many years ago, before he left me and my mother.

To this day, I still can't understand why, but my guilt made him even angrier, "I have to bring you into line. The only thing that will work is to *force* you to be a better wife." Moving toward me, he raised his hand to strike—just as the doorbell rang. I took the opportunity to run into the bedroom and lock the door. Our son, David, was home. It was the distraction Gary needed. There would be no more violence, at least not that night.

The very next day, I discovered the letters. It happened when I was looking for Gary's appointment book to see if he had noted down a doctor's appointment. There they were, clipped together, staring at me from his desk drawer. The first one was postmarked just ten days ago from a city in Gary's sales territory. "My darling Gary," it began, "last night was heaven. I wish I could be holding you now. I miss you more than I know how to say . . ."

It was true. All the fears I'd had over the years were true. Gary didn't love me. Without thinking, I called Gary on the phone and began screaming at him about the letters. I can't even remember what he said because I began to feel so panicky. It was getting hard to breathe—so I hung up, threw on my coat, and drove the few blocks to my friend Maggie's house, hoping she would be there. She was.

"I always knew I would find the evidence one day," I began, too upset to remember to say hello. "How could I have fooled myself for so long? Lots of things are falling into place—the times when he came home a day later than he planned, all his excuses, and the whiff of another woman I sometimes thought came to bed with him. All that interest in the way he dressed, the way his hair was cut. It was for other women, not for me. What an idiot I am!"

I didn't have it in me to stay angry for long. Soon I was blaming myself. "What did I do wrong?" I cried to Maggie. "It must be my fault. I know he's a good man underneath it all. And I need him. How can I live without him? I can't. I know I can't. Oh God, I'd be better off dead."

"Slow down," Maggie urged. "Maybe this is a good thing; maybe this is your opportunity to leave him. Every time we get together you tell me how mean he is to you, Kate, and that he hits you. How long are you going to put up with it? This isn't good for you, or for David. Please think about leaving him. We've known each other for a long time, and I care about you a lot. It upsets me to see you so upset. You deserve better!"

I knew Maggie didn't like Gary. I had shared too many of my troubles with her too often, so she didn't know the good side of him. And she had every right to be frustrated with me; even then I knew I was letting Gary dominate me. I just didn't know I could stop it. Seeing how I turned my eyes away, she cried, *"Listen to me, Kate! You've got to get some help."*

It was as though I had cotton batting in my ears; I could barely hear what she said. That, in itself, scared me. So I threw on my coat and ran out the front door, explaining over my shoulder that I had to pull my thoughts together. My house was quiet when I returned; there was nothing to distract me, no one to ask me to stop and think. It wasn't long before I put my toothbrush and some underwear into a bag, grabbed my checkbook, and took off again in the car.

Several miles from home I realized David would be getting out of school fairly soon, and there was no one there to welcome him. I didn't turn around. "I'm not much of a mother anyway," I heard myself say. "David will do better without me. Nobody really needs me. Mom will cry, but only for a little while. Gary won't shed a tear, he'll be too busy with his girlfriend."

Suddenly I was at that underpass I knew so well, where the road narrowed and veered sharply to the left between stone pillars that supported the bridge above. Through my tears I saw the truck in front of me slow down. Its red brake lights went on. Realizing I was going too fast, I tried to slow down, but my foot seemed frozen. I couldn't make it move toward the brake pedal. Then I felt the car swerve and heard myself scream as the world turned black.

Several days later I woke up in a hospital bed with a serious concussion, a fractured hip, and multiple contusions. Even though I hurt all over, I felt strangely relieved. The accident gave me the respite I needed. For now at least, I was the one who came first. And Gary was at my side, crying and apologetic.

"I swear the affair is over," he offered, tears running down his cheeks. "I know I've lied to you and been unkind to you, but I really love you. I don't understand what gets into me sometimes. I find myself doing things I really don't want to do. I can't help it. Please forgive me. I promise I'll do better. I promise. Just get well."

Gary was almost out of his mind with guilt. He kept saying the problem was his, that he couldn't get his mind off other women. He confessed to believing he was fated to destroy any love that came his way. "I don't want to hurt you, Kate, you know I don't, but something grabs hold of me and I have no control over it. Maybe now, though, after this accident, things will change. I'll make it up to you. Just wait and see."

It didn't matter what he said. Lying in that hospital bed, I wasn't sure I could believe him anyway. And besides, I wasn't feeling much of anything. Nor would I for quite a while. It took several months for my body to heal, but even after that, I was stuck in the mechanics of life. I shudder when I think about it. There was no zest to me, no spice. And my mind was struck dumb. I just stopped thinking. I felt no resentment, but I also had no desire to please Gary. Nothing held my attention—no book, no conversation, no movie, nothing. Once home from the hospital, I spent all my time flat in bed counting the cracks in the ceiling. Even David, my little boy, seemed far away. I ate a little, slept a little, and never cried. The letters had pushed me toward ending my life, and in my own way, I did.

Gary tried to talk to me, he made me food, brought me flowers. He even got angry and yelled at me. But neither presents nor threats raised a spark. I was barely aware of his presence. This was more than he could bear; later he told me it terrified him. So the time finally came when he began to blame me again. I remember him standing at the foot of our bed and saying, "The affair was your fault. If you were there for me, I wouldn't have needed her. If you took care of your body and kept the house better, I wouldn't have been so turned off. But we can do better. I know it. We'll work together on it. Just cooperate. Get your breasts fixed and everything will be all right. You'll see."

I could only nod. Maybe it was all my fault, maybe I should get my breasts fixed. But what difference did it make? There was nothing I could do about it. I didn't care. I was too weary. And so the days wore on slowly, dully.

One day Maggie took me to see Barbara, her therapist. Because Maggie was such a good friend, I didn't object to going. But I also didn't quite know why she was bothering to take me—or why she cared about me so much. I was almost mute during the session. I remember Barbara asking me a question that I couldn't find the energy to answer. Thankfully, that didn't seem to bother her; instead, she said I didn't have to talk and asked if I would like a cup of hot tea and a cookie. I accepted with a nod. Mostly, Barbara and Maggie talked.

And so my therapy began. At first, I brought David with me. I thought therapy would be good for him. Then I began to go alone. Barbara seemed to be on my side, and I liked that. Soon I began to take the antidepressant medication that had been prescribed when I was in the hospital.

Late one afternoon, maybe six months later, and after I had begun therapy, I discovered something very important. When I heard Gary turning the key to come into the house, I felt my body try to get up to greet him while my head couldn't make it off the pillow. I actually was aware that I felt annoyed. And I heard a voice inside saying *NO!* I remember thinking how strange it was that I had never heard that *no* before.

Something was going on inside. Not that anything else changed; mostly I daydreamed and read. If I thought at all, it followed the same old formula: *One day, after I get well, I'll be able to make him love me. I'll listen to him, do what he says, and he won't leave.* But increasingly I was also aware of the voice inside that said *NO!* I couldn't deny the energy that came with it. Even my pulse quickened. I would hear myself say *I can't be as awful as he makes me out to be; I have friends who actually like me.* I began to feel anger, not the kind of anger that disappears in the next moment, but the kind that simmers day in and day out.

I never did get back to making dinner for Gary. It was easier to take David out for a hamburger.

One day Maggie came over and we chatted about her daughter Kerry, who was thirteen and just beginning to get interested in boys. Maggie was trying to get her to put as much into her schoolwork as she used to, and that wasn't easy. It struck me that I was cheering Maggie on! My God, it felt good being able to support her. I was actually getting better.

Soon we got to talking about Gary, and Maggie once again asked why I was still living with him. Much to my surprise, I answered, "I'm not sure why I'm here or whether it's permanent. I used to believe I couldn't make it *without* him, but recently I've figured out how terribly frightened I am of living *with* him."

This reminded me of the time when my father left home, so I told Maggie how he ran away with another woman the night before my tenth birthday. "I woke up expecting a present and instead he was gone. For years I thought he left because I did something terribly wrong. I used to keep his picture on my dresser, and every night I would tell him I was sorry for what I did. Then I would kiss him before climbing into bed."

Maggie seemed interested, so the words continued to spill out. "I was seventeen when I met Gary, and he was twenty-two. He was a waiter and I was a busgirl at a hotel on the Cape. You should have seen us, we

were quite a pair . . . sexy! Everyone was jealous. We would sun ourselves in lounge chairs and parade around the hotel's swimming pool in
our bathing suits. Everything was great until a friend told me Gary was
hanging out with the hotel secretary during my work shift. At first I
didn't want to believe it; in fact, I got angry at her for saying it. But later
I actually saw the two of them whispering to each other. When I asked
Gary about it, he claimed she was just a friend. To this day, I remember
him reassuring me, 'It's you I love, not her.' Ugh! How could I have believed him?

"When I found out she was more than a friend, we went through the
same old routine, though it was new to me at the time. Gary felt guilty
and even cried. He said he never wanted to lose me and promised to be
loyal, but he insisted I let my hair grow long just like hers. Can you
imagine the craziness of it all? I actually had a taste of this year's nightmare way back then when I was seventeen."

It felt good to be talking. "I'm so grateful that my mind is alive again,
Maggie. I'm not so confused. Can you tell?"

Dear friend that she was, Maggie began to cry. "I'm so happy to have
you back. Do you know that you disappeared? I missed you so much."

"I know . . . I know," I replied, crying with her.

Memories kept coming back, things I hadn't thought about for years,
as if I was sorting through my life again. "Did you know, Maggie, that I
wanted to be a doctor? Gary didn't believe I had the head for it. He used
to poke fun at me whenever I brought it up, and I was dumb enough to
forgive him. I thought he was doing it because he was ashamed of his
own poor schoolwork. He couldn't ever get the reading done and his
papers were always late. With some help from me, he finally did gradu-
ate from college, but it took him six years. And I was the one who encouraged him to get a master's degree."

"He actually got that degree," I added wryly, "but I never even applied to medical school."

It took a couple of years for me to get better. I knew it was happening
when the beauty of the tree outside my bedroom window struck me. I
hadn't really seen it for years. And every once in a while I felt my heart

skip a beat when my son laughed. Slowly, I got back into contact with friends, found a job, and even began to argue with Gary. Sometimes he listened patiently, but more often he got angry.

Once, after I complained that he laughed at me in front of others, he got furious. "You're impossible. Can't you take a joke? It's you who's mentally ill, not me!" When I objected, he knocked me across the floor.

That was when I found my angry voice—you might call it my rage. I actually ranted and raved at him over the telephone the next day when he was in another city. And I also found the courage to move out. David, now eleven years old, had been telling me for a long time that he hated the fighting between Gary and me, yet he had begun screaming at me almost as if he were a small rendition of his Dad. And his behavior in school wasn't so good either. So I knew it would be better for both of us if we left. By now, my fear of having to care for David all alone was less daunting. I packed up and left with David while Gary was away on a business trip.

Of course Gary was furious when he found out. One night he knocked on the door to my apartment in a rage, scaring me out of my wits. I'm embarrassed to say that not only did I open the door, I also put a key in his hand. I was too scared to do anything else.

Still, David and I did well. I began to think less about my aging body and more about the world around me. I got a promotion at work. And David's smile grew broader, his play easier, less violent at home.

Then the unthinkable happened. One night about a year after the move, I went to a parent-teacher meeting and met Ken. He wasn't the kind of guy I would have been interested in years ago. He wasn't particularly handsome and he didn't have a lot of money, but he had a sweet smile and a spirited daughter. I liked him. It's hard for me to tell you why, and maybe that doesn't matter, except when he looked into my eyes, I knew it was *me* he was seeing, and he *liked* what he saw.

You would probably find it hard to imagine how deeply surprised I was one night when he asked what I thought about his daughter's poor study habits! I wanted to pinch myself to see if I was dreaming. Gary would never have thought of asking for my advice. Ken, astonished that I had such self-doubt, shook his head in disbelief. I couldn't figure out how I got lucky enough to have such a man walk into my life.

But there was still the specter of Gary to contend with. Even though Ken and I kept our relationship secret, bits of information began to slip out, probably through David. And then Gary dropped by late in the evening and found too many dinner dishes in the sink.

"It was your lover who came for dinner, right?"

When I didn't answer, he attacked: "You're a whore and you know it. You're not telling me the truth. But I still know what you're up to. I'm not a fool. You've always been a liar."

I was shaking inside, but I knew I had to keep my voice clear and strong—not furious but angry. "You don't live here anymore, Gary. We're separated. You have no right to say those things."

"I'll never forgive you for what you've done to me," he yelled, as if what I said about his behavior never registered. "From the moment we met, you were trouble. You've been running around for years."

"Stop it, Gary," I yelled, looking squarely into his eyes. "Get real. Our relationship is over. I don't have any feeling for you anymore. I no longer want you in my life. I'm finished. It's done. And you have to leave the apartment."

Huffing and puffing, he turned around and walked out the door. I was amazed.

Slowly, ever so slowly, we actually tore ourselves away from each other. One day I changed the lock on the door and refused to open it when he came by. And then I stopped answering his telephone calls. Finally, thankfully, the day came when he met another woman. Not that I wasn't jealous. I was. David and I began to see less of him—and I actually felt relieved.

It's now been five full years since I moved out of that beautiful prison I used to call my home. I received my divorce papers just the other day. More and more, I can see how badly Gary treated me—and how I let him do it. I even know why. Meanwhile, I'm continually amazed by Ken and the love we have together. Who would have ever thought I could have a relationship like this? Certainly not me! No one but my dear friend Maggie and my therapist had that faith. I'm so thankful they did.

David is a teenager and he's doing very well. I like his friends. His grades have improved and he doesn't lose his temper in school anymore. It does happen at home, but only now and then. Better still, he talks about it with Ken.

And I no longer live at the edge of anxiety. I shop for clothes, laugh with my friends, get angry at my mother, go to work, and take care of my son. Ken and I make dinner and go to the movies. We get together with friends, we argue, and we make great love. A rather remarkable life for a woman who once chose to die!

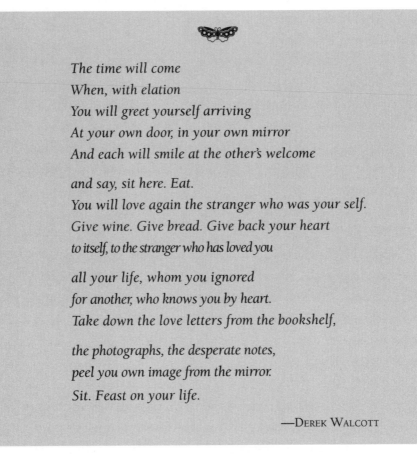

The time will come
When, with elation
You will greet yourself arriving
At your own door, in your own mirror
And each will smile at the other's welcome

and say, sit here. Eat.
You will love again the stranger who was your self.
Give wine. Give bread. Give back your heart
to itself, to the stranger who has loved you

all your life, whom you ignored
for another, who knows you by heart.
Take down the love letters from the bookshelf,

the photographs, the desperate notes,
peel you own image from the mirror.
Sit. Feast on your life.

—DEREK WALCOTT

FINDING THE KEY

There's a tale about an old woman who was out walking late one night when she came upon a girl searching for something under a streetlight.

"What are you looking for?" the old woman asked.

"I'm looking for the key," said the girl.

The old woman joined in the search, but they didn't find it. And so she asked, "Where exactly did you lose the key?"

"Over there," the girl answered, pointing toward a dark doorway about ten feet away.

Confused, the old woman wondered, "If you lost the key over there, why are you looking here?"

And the response came, "This is where the light is."

There should be a warning that screams *danger* when an adolescent girl thinks of herself as a pretty thing, a doll whose reason for being is to please others. And if the problem persists into adulthood, the girl, or someone who loves her, needs to cry out for help. But many people, Kate and her parents included, don't have that awareness; they're caught in the spell cast by the female archetype that prescribes such behavior. So Kate continued for so long to look for love in her old way, under the light, when she needed to look in the darkness of her own psyche. Indeed, that was the only place where she stood a chance of finding it. The problem was, she feared the dark. Her fear was so great that she chose death instead, and when that didn't happen, a deathlike depression.

Create a picture in your mind's eye of a pretty little child, sweet, compliant, and often pampered. As a woman, she's still a child who relies on others to lead her, and given the needs of those others, she might be a sexual object as well. In effect, she's a thing to be indulged, petted, and even abused. That's the effect of a particular female archetype that has so many of us under its spell. It also describes the severely depressed woman named Kate who walked into my office with her friend one day. The dark that she feared inside was her own rage and the emptiness that lay below.

I remember sitting with her in silence, sensing the simmering anger and the heaviness of her body—indeed, of the very air around her. As is my practice in therapy, I placed some awareness in my own mind/body process and looked for my reactions to Kate. I found some of that same heaviness she felt: sadness is often catching. And I felt my own anger. It was a very old anger that had lodged inside me when I was an adolescent trying to find a way out of another rendition of that old female archetype. And here, sitting right before me in my office, was an example in grown-up form. Over the years I have seen many of these women and watched many renditions of their pain and suffering.

It's not as though Kate's parents made a conscious decision to hurt her; like most parents, they wanted only the best for her. However, much parenting is habit-driven, an unconscious pattern that repeats itself from generation to generation. Like her mother before her, Kate's unique personality, her particular temperament, tastes, or curiosity, were tamped down. No one was to blame; her parents knew no other way. At the root of the problem was the difficulty we all have breaking out of habit-driven behavior.

If he were alive today, Martin Buber would call this habit-driven parenting an example of an *I-It* relationship; the word *It* refers to the child being treated as a thing to be used, an object designed to suit her parents or to fulfill the archetype that guided them. Treated as an *It*, a girl doesn't develop a self of her own; she feels empty and so needs others to lead her. But she also resents being led. In this sense, she is angrily addicted to the influence of others.

As an alternative, Martin Buber would suggest *I-Thou* parenting, which assumes a little bit of God in every child, including this girl child named Kate. As a conscious approach to parenting, *I-Thou* suggests that the challenge of parents is to help their child manifest as a singular being, an embodiment of the diversity that characterizes a sacred world.[1]

Kate's silence during the first sessions we spent together gave me the time to travel through thoughts like these. I was also able to find the stillness I needed to be present for her. I knew rather quickly that there was no way to relate to Kate with words; she really couldn't respond in kind at that time. Instead, the challenge was to focus my awareness on her, meeting her eyes when she allowed that to happen, and sometimes smiling my acceptance of her even if she wasn't looking. And we breathed together.

Slowly, ever so slowly, in psychotherapy and with the help of medication, Kate came out of her depression. At first it was a matter of just accomplishing the basics: eating, sleeping, and moving her body several times during the day. Gary took her for a walk every morning and Maggie made food for her. Every afternoon her son played on her bed, whether she was awake or sleeping. At times, when the waves of depression ebbed, she and I explored the story she was living and how it had become another kind of death. But for a long time her world was very dark, and we could do little but wait.

So it was truly a miracle when, at long last, she heard herself say, "*NO*." This was no fleeting sound; it came as a loud, insistent push, much like a surge of electricity. Not only was there something going on inside, but Kate was aware of it. The idea of getting up to greet Gary came with a very clear *NO* in her mind and the powerful surge of an angry feeling in her body. The combination woke her up. Her trouble felt real to her. She couldn't deny the reality that she was furious at her husband.

In therapy, this was the starting point, a foundation from which we could build. Once, when she felt that anger during a session, I asked her to close her eyes and find it in her body. She said it felt like a searing pain in her chest. As part of the process, I then suggested she keep her awareness trained on that pain, watching for some change, be it in location, in intensity, or even in quality—it could even change into some other feeling. Indeed, that's what happened. After a while, the searing pain in her chest faded and a certain kind of flutter emerged in her stomach. That was fear. It was a fear of Gary, certainly, but as we soon learned, it was also a fear of her own emptiness, that gnawing hole she felt inside her stomach. This was a significant step on the path toward healing.

Imagine being in a serious depression. On the continuum of awareness, this is at the very low end. Thinking is confined to the concrete, the tangible. The world is gray and feelings are blunted. Life contracts to the most minimal of repetitive behaviors. No sunset, no baby's smile, not even a lover can hold one's attention. When Kate was seriously depressed, she didn't experience any mood or emotion, and there was nothing much to think about.

Only a little higher on the continuum is what we call being on automatic. Within this state, much of life is made up of habitual behavior.

Getting up, brushing our teeth, going to work are all accomplished with very little awareness. Sometimes summers come and go, babies are born, grow up, leave the house, and we're barely aware of it. Kate was on automatic when she lived with Gary. Even her complaining was habitual; it had no energy behind it. She forgot about it in the next moment. Most of us get lost in automatic living for periods of time during every single day.

At the high end of the continuum of awareness are those exquisite moments when we are experiencing *focused* or *one-pointed* awareness. We really *see* the baby's smile, *hear* her laugh, *feel* her tiny heart beat, *taste* the sweetness of her new skin. When this happens, time itself slows down. Experiences like these become high points in life. As Kate moved out of her depression, she had moments when the trees outside her window caught her attention, her son's laughter opened her heart, and she could receive Ken's love.

Given where we are on that continuum, our six senses (seeing, hearing, tasting, smelling, feeling, and, in meditation, thinking) take in more or less information. At one end of the continuum, it's as though our eyeglasses are dirty, so very little information gets in. Somewhere in the middle, our glasses become cleaner, and we experience more of life. But it's still minimal; new information has to be very intense to grab our attention. At the other end, with new glasses, it's possible to see very clearly. The world becomes brighter, more alive. With heightened states of awareness, not just sight but all our senses are open and vibrating.[2]

We can all increase our capacity for one-pointed awareness. It can help us know our emotions. For this work, it's helpful to realize that emotions are composed of both thoughts in the mind and feelings in the body. Knowing both is important, because thoughts by themselves can be thoroughly confusing, while feelings in the body tend to be grounding. Stub your toe, and you know for sure that it hurts; think about stubbing your toe, and you might hear yourself drown in self-blame. *I should have watched where I was going. Why am I so clumsy?* If this happens, the pain in your stubbed toe can get so scrambled with your blaming mind that you end up in a muddle.

Being aware of the difference between feelings in the body and thoughts in the mind is certainly valuable, but being grounded in feelings as they are expressed in the body is priceless. By way of example, Kate's awareness of the *NO* she felt in her body when Gary came home became a touchstone. Over time she realized that her *NO* emerged rather frequently when Gary was around, and that she got angry in response to his abusive behavior. Then she became aware of the fear that came along with her *NO*.

Now Kate could name her trouble: she was in an abusive relationship. And she could name two of the emotions her trouble triggered: anger and fear. All this existed. It was real. Of that she was sure.

There are less dramatic ways to gain insight into your emotions. You can observe yourself watching television or a movie. Notice, for instance, what happens when you're watching a horror film. Do your muscles feel tense? Focus on that tension and ask yourself, *Am I afraid? Am I angry? Is it a combination of the two?* You can also ask, *Is this muscle tension constant, or does it change as the music changes?*

Watch your body while looking at a news report on terror. Perhaps you'll detect a flicker of discomfort in your stomach. What word would you use to label the feeling? Is it fear? Is it anxiety? Does it go away after the show is over, or does it hang around and enter into your dreams at night? These are experiments that ask you to use awareness to learn more about your own particular body sensations.

A greater awareness of the body sensations that are part of an emotion can help you feel centered in your own experience. Then it's easier to act on your own behalf. For Kate, it was a first step toward the dissolution of a bad marriage. And then she found another man to love. It appears that her story therefore has a happy ending. Instead, I would say it has a happy intermission. She came a long way from being a woman who tried to kill herself to the vibrant woman she is now. Questions still remain: Will she stay on the path toward wholeness, or is Ken the next man in whom she will lose herself? At the end of the story she tells, Kate is optimistic about her future; unfortunately, it may also be that she is still looking in the wrong place for the key to her happiness.

Nevertheless, Kate found her way out of a deep depression, left an abusive marriage, reared a thriving child, and found someone who could love her. Each is evidence of the strength this woman found in herself and predictive of the good things to come in the future. Kate is on the path to wholeness and still has a way to go.

In the following meditation you will again bring your awareness to the body. Now, body sensations come in many forms. Broadly speaking, we can separate them into two categories: *physiologically* based sensations, such as the touch of the air against your skin or the rhythm of your heartbeat, and *psychologically* based sensations, such as the muscle tightness that often accompanies anger or the tears that accompany sadness.

My teacher, Shinzen, suggests that we call body sensations that are primarily physiologically based *external touch* and body sensations that are primarily psychologically based *internal feel*. If you sense the touch of your clothes on your thigh, or the sensation of skin touching skin, that's external touch. This category also includes sensations that are deeply embedded in physiology, such as the sensation of your ribs expanding as air fills up your lungs or the rhythmical beat of your heart.

On the other hand, if you sense a flutter in your abdomen or tension in your jaw, that's likely to be internal feel. These are the body sensations that, together with thought, make up our emotions or moods. For example, you may feel heat arise in your face when you're angry at your child. At the same time, you may also be aware of irate thoughts. Both the feeling in your body and the thoughts in your mind make up the emotion called anger.[3]

Locating body sensations helps us be clear about what we feel. External touch sensations, such as an itch or a pain, have locations. So does a pulse. Internal feel sensations, such as sadness or anger, also have locations, but many tend to be felt in the face or along the front of the torso. A headache or a flutter in the stomach are two examples. And of course, while there are common locations for internal feel, as individuals we also feel in our own idiosyncratic ways.

With awareness we also become aware of the *impermanence* of bodily sensations. While some emotions appear to be stable, with awareness we learn that all emotions arise, have their moment in time, and fall away. Even the most stable of moods doesn't last forever. Knowing the fleeting nature of an emotion can give us the patience to live it inside ourselves rather than out in the interpersonal world. That's a special kind of freedom!

The following meditation is designed to help you practice being aware of body sensations. Using a meditative technique called *free-floating awareness*, you will let your awareness land where it likes, keeping track as it moves from one place in the body to the next. The challenge is to let your awareness arise and fade by itself, without any interference.

I'll ask you to label out loud the place where your awareness lands. So, for instance, if it lands on your knees, you say "knees." Labeling is a way of strengthening your capacity for sustained concentration. If it works for you, use it. If not, let it go. In any case, stay with each body sensation until another takes its place. Please feel free to put down the book or push the pause on your CD player so you can extend the time of meditation a little longer. Also, remember to be as curious as a natural scientist observing the flight of a hawk or the bubbling of a chemical reaction. If you can take the stance of an observer, you'll interfere less with the flow of information from your senses.

When it's convenient, find a quiet place and a straight-backed chair or a cushion. If you like, use the memory prompt that's outlined in the summary at the end of the meditation. And keep a paper and pencil handy, because it can be helpful to record what has happened. Now . . . settle in.

I do not know which to prefer
The beauty of inflection
Or the beauty of innuendo

The black bird singing
Or just after

—Wallace Stevens

A Meditation on Cultivating Awareness

Close your eyes, and feel your body hanging on your spine. Relax into the body and take a few deep breaths. Now repeat the meditation called "A Meditation on Finding the Stillness" that appears at the end of chapter 1. Be aware.

❁

When you're ready, make the object of your awareness **external touch***. Let your awareness float freely through the body. Perhaps it will settle on your feet where they touch the floor . . . on your chest where it touches your shirt . . . on your face where the air brushes your skin. You might sense your hands as they rest on your thighs . . . your eyelids where they touch each other.*

Label out loud each time your awareness shifts, feet . . . chest . . . face . . . hands . . . eyelids.

Your awareness might land on a pang of hunger that arises in the stomach . . . label that stomach*. Your awareness might land on a feeling of sleepiness that fills the whole body . . . label that* whole body*. And give the permission to be.*

You might miss a lot of available sensations . . . but that's okay . . . this is a beginning. Over time you'll be aware of more.

If a thought arises, make it background. This means, note that it's there. Thoughts will continue to arise and fade . . . be aware and gently return to the body.

Set your timer for five minutes, and let your awareness float freely among these various kinds of external touch.

❁

After five minutes have passed, shift the object of your meditation to **internal feel***. Let your awareness land on those places in your body where you experience moods or emotions . . . joy . . . excitement . . . anger . . . sadness . . . impatience . . .*

Start with your face. Perhaps the small muscles around your eyes are tense . . . if so, label that eyes*. Notice that tenseness until your awareness is pulled somewhere else.*

Continue with your throat as well as your face. Maybe your awareness will land on a lump you feel in your throat and the tears that fall from your eyes. Label that throat and eyes. *And watch with curiosity . . . with interest in your body's capacity to express feeling.*

Then explore your chest and your abdomen. Are there flickers of sensation that you might call fear in your chest? Label that chest.

You might feel the kind of nervousness that makes you want to jump out of your skin . . . and it's all over your body. Label that all over.

And if there's an absence of feeling, label that none.

Whatever feelings arise . . . anger . . . sadness . . . jealousy . . . pleasure . . . happiness . . . peace . . . pour acceptance and love into them all. Watch as they arise, manifest, and fade. This is equanimity, a balanced mind, not preferring one or feeling over another. Sense each one . . . and be aware.

Set your timer for ten minutes and let your awareness float freely through the body . . . observing **internal feel.**

❦

Now, shift your awareness so that it includes **external touch** *and* **internal feel.** *In effect, be aware of any body sensation that arises. Try to catch as many as you can and label their location.*

Set your timer and take another ten minutes to watch. You might think of your awareness as a butterfly . . . alighting on one or another body sensation.

❦

After the ten minutes, slowly open your eyes. Sit quietly for a while and let the light shine in. Now . . . in the quiet . . . recall the trouble you named during the first meditation . . . and be aware of any **internal feel** *body sensations that arise.*

If you feel nothing, that's all right. Simply enjoy the peace that your body is offering. And label that nothing.

If you feel a heaviness all over the body and you associate it with sadness, label that all over. *If you feel flutters in your abdomen, label that* abdomen. *Remember, you don't have to be right or even accurate.*

If, instead . . . as you hold your trouble in your mind . . . the muscles in your body relax and you're filled with relief, you now know that, when confronted by trouble, you're likely to feel relieved if you face it. This is an **insight** *that might help in your effort to heal the emotions.*

Whatever your reaction, whether it's clarity . . . confusion . . . insight . . . or no reaction at all . . . be aware . . . matter-of-fact. And if your reactions are too upsetting . . . if you can't be matter-of-fact . . . you might want to enlist the aid of a trained counselor or a meditation coach who can help you pursue this path.

❀

When you're ready . . . let go of trouble as an object of meditation . . . and spend several minutes dwelling in the meditation called "A Meditation on Finding the Stillness." This will help calm the mind/body process. Then end the meditation by writing down what you have learned. And please remember, there is no correct outcome to meditation. Everything is information.

May all beings know awareness.

Training for Awareness

1. Repeat "A Meditation on Finding the Stillness."

2. Let your awareness float freely through the body, labeling the location of sensations called **external touch**.

3. Let your awareness float freely through those parts of the body where you can sense **internal feel**. Label the locations.

4. Let your awareness float freely through the body. Be aware of **external touch** and **internal feel**. Label the locations.

5. Recall the trouble you named in the last meditation and be aware of **internal feel**. Label the locations.

Three

Sex, Fantasy, and a Married Woman Named Laura

It was an afternoon fit for loving. A coral color tipped the high cirrus clouds as they crept slowly across the sky, a light breeze cooled the skin, and gently rolling waves emptied the mind. From my patch of blanket, I could see a woman far down the beach running toward me at the water's edge; her arms and legs moved with such grace that each leap seemed effortless. Wisps of the surf's foam rose up around her feet, and the setting sun caressed her body. The entire world was aglow and my runner shimmered within it.

The closer she came, the more enthralled I became. Soon I could see how her bathing suit streamlined her torso while leaving the muscles in her legs free to ripple. Her long black hair was tied in a tail that swung rhythmically side to side. She was like a magnificent cat, curiously still even as she moved.

Nearby, a lone couple sat nestled in each other's arms. They turned their heads to watch her; I could see that they, too, were captured by her beauty. Flickers of jealousy rose within me, and I began to think of ways to distract their attention, but soon the man turned away, downing his lust with a swallow of beer. The woman's gaze lingered a little longer, as she slowly drizzled grains of sand down the calf of her lover's leg.

Can you imagine my excitement when the runner slowed down and stopped at the water's edge, right there in front of me? How thrilling it was to see her raise her arms high, her body open and accepting, as she dove into each swell. I watched as each wave broke and swept her back to me inside its foam. Finally, she collapsed in abandon at the water's edge.

Then I took a risk that was so unlike me it verged on the unbelievable. I rose from my blanket and, with each step more deliberate than the last, approached her prone body. She was like some strange force that had the power to draw me ever closer. Now I could see crystals of water trembling on her belly. Too frightened to move any nearer, I bent down on my haunches and watched a small hermit crab surface from the froth near her toes and quickly scurry away, dragging his secondhand home behind. Bubbles broke on the sand, and rivulets of water made long runs as though gently scratching the back of a lover.

Opening her eyes, she looked up at me and smiled a yes to the question I didn't have the nerve to ask. So I stretched out on the sand next to her and carefully, tenderly, traced the outline of her cheekbones with my forefinger. Her eyes were my ocean, deep blue with sunlight sparkling on the surface. Falling into those eyes, I sensed the beat of our hearts and the ebb and flow of the ocean.

Just as I was about to lean over and kiss her, a troubling roar rolled out of the distance. Try as I might, I couldn't ignore it. I had to open my eyes. That's when I realized I was lying in bed next to my husband, Ned, and the TV was on. He was in his shorts with two or three pillows supporting his head and a can of beer in his hand. The U.S. Open was proceeding full force, and the roar was coming from the crowd's enthusiastic applause.

For a moment I wasn't sure which scene was real—the image of my runner lying at the water's edge or the bedroom with Ned and the television. Past my toes, however, I could see the chaos of creams and makeup, money, keys, and receipts on top of my dresser. The things were all too clear, the heavy burgundy draperies all too suffocating.

Frustrated, uncomfortably at loose ends, I squeezed my eyelids shut and determined to return to my runner. But no matter how hard I tried, I couldn't find her. She was gone. The effort evoked an old and frightening emptiness in the pit of my stomach—along with a fierce desire for sex. What was I doing fantasizing about a woman when I had my husband in bed with me?

With surprise I heard myself think, *But I don't want him.* And then, *Who do I want? What's wrong with me? Am I a lesbian, just like my daughter, Jeanie?*

Realizing I was awake, Ned shifted his attention away from the television and began teasing me in that slightly mocking tone of his, always a cue that he was angry. "The greatest match of the season and you don't even notice. Here you are, Laura, lying in bed right in front of the TV, and you might as well be a thousand miles away."

His sarcasm woke me up. "This *is* my reality," I thought, "so I'd better pay attention." But he had already turned back to the game as if there was nothing else to say. Neither of us was any good at being angry. Ned usually made one or two sarcastic comments and then beat a fast retreat. I was no different; it was rare for me to stand up for myself, and that usually came with a river of tears. But this was certainly not the moment for me to try to do anything different. I wanted to sort things out, and for that to happen there had to be peace in the house. So I ignored Ned's sarcasm and tried to change the subject: "Why was the crowd so excited?"

His retort was quick and sharp: "You spend the entire evening sleeping or daydreaming or whatever it is you do, and then you expect me to believe you want to know about the game? Give me a break. Go back to your studio and work on your documentary. That holds your attention. Or go back to sleep; you probably find that more interesting too."

I needed no further permission. Now I could leave. Without another word, I threw on my bathrobe, went downstairs, and sank into my thoughts about Jeanie and me. She was nineteen and in her second year of college. Our only child, she was as smart as both of us put together and prettier than I ever was. I recalled how my heart had almost burst with pride when she had given the valedictorian speech at her high school graduation. And I was thankful for the times when she read her poetry to me. It was witty and insightful. She was a young woman of many talents.

How lonely the house was when she first went away! But this, her second year at college, was different, maybe because there was time to work on the documentary about sick kids I had contracted to do for a TV special. It helped that Jeanie was busy and happy, and I knew that even though we didn't talk much, when something important came up she would call. I did hear about her roommates, her courses, and the teachers she liked and didn't like. I must admit, though, we never really got personal, she and I. Something kept us apart. I always thought it was my discomfort with people, even my own daughter.

She had told me me that she was a lesbian at least a month ago, but it was more of a report than a sharing. And, I realized, this was information I really didn't want to have. Jeanie had tried all sorts of things over the years, only to drop them. There was her dramatic phase, as Ned and I called it, when she was sure she would become an actress. Then there was her medical phase, when she swore she'd be a surgeon. Maybe her lover, Ruth, was just another one of those phases. That's why I never told Ned—and because I knew it would upset him.

So when Jeanie and Ruth actually came into town and made their announcement over dinner last weekend, it came as something of a surprise, even for me. Ned, to his credit, was polite and even tactful with the girls. Only later, when we were alone, did he let me know how confused and hurt he felt. "Did I do something wrong? Was I a bad father?" And, after some silence, "If she's really serious, we'll never have grandchildren."

I tried to console him, but I'd never been much good at that. Besides, I was preoccupied with my own fears. I worried that Jeanie would notice how hard it was for me to look straight into her eyes, or even talk with her. Ned stayed away; he had work to do. Finally the girls left, and we breathed a sigh of relief.

However, for me the relief didn't last for long. Jeanie and Ruth were a puzzle that kept bothering me. I couldn't stop thinking about it. After all, I tried to reason with myself, Jeanie was a grown-up. She had the right to make her own choices. That, in fact, is what I had said to her on the telephone just a few days ago: "All I want is for you to be happy, and if this is what will do it, that's fine." I really did believe what I said, but it didn't quite match what I felt.

Now, in the middle of the night a full week later, lying on the couch in the living room with a picture of baby Jeanie on the piano, I couldn't help wondering if I was responsible for Jeanie's preference. Wasn't my dream evidence of it? Had I been hiding my preference for women throughout my married life? Was I being unfair to Ned?

I loved Ned. He was a good man, even if sarcastic at times. Our sex life had been mostly satisfying to both of us. Sure, we went through some bad times—my miscarriage and his affair—but we came through them. More and more, in recent years, I understood how important he was to me. We lived our lives in tandem, and Ned was the one I wanted to comfort me, the one I wanted to understand me. But the question remained: was I sexually attracted to him or was our lovemaking just a sham?

It was so confusing. I could barely stand thinking about it. Suddenly, without even being aware of my intention, I found myself walking down the hall and actually getting back into bed with Ned. I wanted to forget about Jeanie's announcement. I had to be close to Ned to feel better.

But he was still annoyed. "Are you going to sleep?" he asked. "Where do you want to be, at home or on some exotic adventure? Tell me and maybe I'll go, too."

"Let's not make a big deal over what happened earlier," I retorted. "The game bored me, so I fell asleep. That's it. There's nothing more to say."

Internally I shuddered at the lie, at my defensiveness. How could I be so dishonest? Why did he put up with me? So I tried again and did a little better, but still I avoided the full truth. "You're right, all this napping and daydreaming isn't good. Even the mystery stories I love to read are bad. They keep me in my own world. But you know that I've always lived inside my head."

He was listening, so I continued: "Even as a child, I liked to be alone. I remember sitting upstairs in my bedroom dressing my dolls and trying to avoid my parents' guests. Of course, if I came down, my mother would make some unkind remark about how I did my hair or the clothes I wore. She always thought there was something wrong with me. I guess I thought so, too. And when I was a teenager I spent most of my time reading one novel after another. Maybe I was avoiding my parents. Maybe I simply preferred my own company."

All these words made the space between us friendlier, so I moved close enough to feel his leg alongside mine. I wanted to break through the distance between us, and I found the courage to ask for it: "I need to be close to you. Let's make love."

But Ned was still too hurt. "Not now," he said gruffly. "We speak so little most of the time that I feel alone even when you begin to talk. Sometimes I think we're like two cats, living in the same house, but so solitary, so afraid to be close. The image troubles me. Go to sleep. We'll make love another time."

Still, we cuddled spoon fashion, and I could feel the touch of his skin and the warmth of his breath on my neck. When we held each other like this I knew that somehow we would be all right. I wished I was a better mate to him and even let myself think that maybe I could be. Soon my body relaxed and I began to feel sleepy.

How confusing it was when, in the midst of these warm fuzzy feelings toward Ned, my runner returned! There was no way I could resist the roundness of her, the way her breasts welcomed me. The fullness of her hips was clearer, more revealed than everyday life ever allowed. The image drew me like the taste of bittersweet chocolate.

When Ned fell asleep I was once again alone with my secret life. Why was it so compelling? Did my daughter grow up having secrets like that? Did she catch it from me? Or maybe she was braver.

I was so uncomfortable with myself I could barely stand it. I had to do something. I decided to see Barbara, a therapist referred to me by a friend. But I was very clear with her: my therapy had to be a secret; I would not tell my husband—or any of my friends. Even with that understanding, I'm such a private person that being in therapy was hard for me. I didn't want Barbara to make me into something—my mother had done enough of that. So I stayed wary, but not so wary that I didn't tell my story. As I think about it, I must have trusted her more than I thought, because I didn't hide anything. And that helped.

I told Barbara about my mother and her friend Julia, when they were young and I was still a child. The two women were an unusual pair. Julia was pretty, almost a fantasy with her golden hair and gentle voice. A free spirit, she was in love with her piano. In contrast, my mother was a hardworking housewife who presided like a grim servant over her kitchen and her children. She was caught in the mechanics of life, except when it came to Julia, whom she indulged with the food she served, the clothes she altered, and the careful way she manicured her nails.

And Julia indulged my mother. She came to our house almost every afternoon for a cup of coffee and a chat. I can still remember the sound of my mother's voice as she confided to her friend about her husband. "He's never happy. You should have heard how he complained about the salad I made for him last night. I know he doesn't like salads, but he has to lose some weight. I don't know what to do anymore. He's just impossible."

"Don't be so hard on him. He was probably in a bad mood," her friend replied, ever the peacemaker.

They had their secret world, these two women. Often they went to the movies—sorry, that's not quite right, they went to see *films*.

Julia chose them after reading reviews in the *New York Times*. I remember that once she even convinced my mother to go to a poetry reading. When I came home that afternoon, they were both excitedly reading Kahlil Gibran to each other. It was a side of them no one else knew about. The two women lived to be old. Julia died first; my mother went soon after.

For as long as she lived, Julia was patient with me, always ready to listen to a story about school or a friend, always interested in teaching me how to do my hair or play the piano. She also protected me from my mother's wrath. I dreamed of growing up to be just like her.

Julia was married to George, a cross between a bodybuilder and a philosopher. He was a cynic, a man who was angry at the world. My father liked George. They spent lots of time together grumbling about life. But there's a difference between spending time together and being close. I learned early that the men were outsiders, loners brushing past each other over dinner or before the TV. Never did they get together without the women. And they didn't know any of the really important information about our world: my mother's friend Sarah's abortion, for instance, or Jessie's divorce. Even Uncle Henry's cancer was kept secret from them. No one told me either, but I listened closely.

Somehow Julia and my mother made things go smoothly on Sundays when everyone got together. Friends and family came to our semi-attached house on a tree-lined street in Flatbush because it was big enough to hold everyone. There was even a little garden in front and a place to sit and watch the neighbors walk by. One particular Sunday stands out because I saw something that puzzled me and heard something else that I kept secret through all the years.

"Hurry, hurry," my mother snarled as she burst into my room early that morning. "You have to help me clean the house. Dust the furniture. Set the table. Why do you always forget to put away your clothes? I'm going to tell Julia," she threatened.

"All right, all right," I responded grumpily as I tried to open my eyes to the morning light. I put away my clothes, made my bed, vacuumed the floors, and dusted all the small turns and knobs on the dining room table, wishing once again that my mother liked modern furniture. Meanwhile I waited for Julia and, with somewhat less pleasure, George. Even my father waited—in the garden or down in the basement—away from my mother's anxious demands.

Finally, they arrived. And I braced myself for George's usual clumsy hello. "Hi kid, you're looking awfully pretty," he said, giving me a bear hug, a tweak of the cheek, and a silver dollar. My head down, I studied the floor and wondered again how Julia could stand him.

"Not so pretty, and especially not so smart," my mother complained, her voice loud as she emphasized the word *smart*. "The only way I could get her to clean her room this morning was to say you and Julia were coming."

Julia interrupted quietly but firmly. "Both pretty and smart. That's who she is, whether she cleans or not."

Tears came to my eyes as I remembered her words.

Soon they all began to talk about the news of the week, and I retreated to the stairs that led up to the second floor, ever ready to scoot up to my bedroom if I had to. Then came dinner, and the refrain of comments about my mother's food. Dad was ever quick to criticize: "This roast is overdone. What's wrong with this applesauce?" Our guests were quick to make up for him with compliments: "You've outdone yourself this time; the cherry filling is perfect." I hated the food. It was boring.

Dad was usually the first to move toward the living room and his favorite chair. Soon the other men followed. The women stayed in the kitchen. I was still young enough to move freely between the two groups but really didn't feel welcome in either. Hovering as unobtrusively as possible, I listened to the men talk about the war. It was a mystery, all this imagery of men with guns, airplanes with bombs. And I stood at the door to the kitchen, overhearing the women complaining in muted voices about the men—another mystery.

At last my father got tired of the conversation about which side was winning and trumpeted toward the kitchen, "Julia, how about a song on the accordion?" She came in obligingly, quickly, and settled herself in a straight-backed chair. The accordion always seemed too big for her. My father folded his hands on his rather round stomach and smiled contentedly. The dishes finally done, my mother sat across the room from him.

Julia urged me to sit next to her, at the same time whispering into my ear, "And you, my dear, are a jewel. Trust in that and let yourself shine."

I wanted nothing more than to be with her.

Night came and everyone left. My parents were actually patient with each other as they put things away. They even kissed me good night. I watched from my bed as my mother stroked my father's balding head and led him into the bedroom. "Come, it's time to go to sleep."

Snuggling under the covers, my world felt perfect. The war was too far away to worry about, and who could ask for a better family? And Julia was my favorite person.

However, I woke up in the middle of the night with a bad stomachache. And my head hurt. I thought of calling out to my mother, but I imagined her putting the light on and asking me anxious questions, so I decided to manage the cramps by myself. When they got really bad, I made my way to the bathroom.

Passing the closed door to my parents' bedroom, I heard strange sounds. Curious and a little worried, I thought about calling out and asking if everything was all right. Instead, I opened the door a crack. My parents were moving in an embrace I couldn't quite understand but somehow knew was private. And then I heard my mother cry out, "Julia . . . Julia . . ." I scurried away and hid under my covers.

The scene was confusing and—for reasons I didn't understand—embarrassing, so I never mentioned it to anyone. Actually, I did such a good job of keeping silent that the memory didn't even surface until late that very night while I was lying in bed next to my husband. My parents' sexuality came as a happy surprise. I was glad they could be intimate, given how much they argued. But what did Julia have to do with it? Waking up the next morning entwined with Ned's body, the question simmered with still another one that my therapist kept asking: "Why do I need my hidden life?"

What, I wondered, would Julia advise? The answer came quickly: "You're a jewel, Laura. Trust in that and let yourself shine."

A warm glow spread through my body, just as it had so long ago. I felt held in her love. In her arms, I could even love myself. And so I decided to come out of hiding.

"Ned," I said as he stirred, "I have something to share with you. It's a story, a fantasy. Would you like to hear it?"

"Yes," he said in a sleepy voice. "I would."

And so I returned to my runner, only this time with Ned. There was a moment right after I began when he held his breath and paused, as if trying to decide whether or not to be upset. It was brief. Fortunately, our excitement carried the day. "Yes, go on," he said. "I have fantasies, too."

"She's running down the beach almost in slow motion . . . her body is silky and taut . . . soon she's close enough for us to hear her panting, see the blue of her eyes and the softness of her smile . . . she's open and accepting of us . . . it's almost as though we are *her* fantasy . . . and then we lie down at the water's edge . . ."

Ned and I kissed deeply as the image of my runner's eyes and the feel of our bodies melted into each other, and we were all carried away on waves of desire.

When the ocean surges
Let me not just hear it

Let it splash within my chest!

—RUMI

WHO AM I?

Things had not gone well for Laura since early adolescence. She was tucked away inside herself, separated from others by a wall of distraction. Yet because she had such a remarkable talent for life, I knew that if she found a way out of herself, the gifts she would bring back to the rest of us would be rich.

So what was her trouble? We could say it was the relationship with her husband. We could also say it was her mother. Certainly her sexual orientation was troubling her. And let's not forget our culture's rigid sexual code, which made loving herself as a woman attracted to women very difficult. Laura was also clearly upset about her daughter's lifestyle. Meanwhile, she was facing the reality of her aging. We might then conclude that all these issues were involved. But it was more than the issues themselves; her very *self*, more accurately her *selves*, were creating trouble.

Laura had an inner voice that criticized her harshly. There was also a small child inside who felt terribly unloved and demeaned. And she had a dreamer inside who conjured up the loving woman she craved but could not, would not, have. Maybe hardest of all was a self that was embarrassed most of the time.

Not that this was all of Laura; she was also a gardener, a filmmaker, a mother, a wife, a friend, and a cook. She was a colleague, an artist, and a devotee of good literature. "I am large, I contain multitudes," Walt Whitman said more than a hundred years ago. From the perspective of Mindfulness Psychotherapy, we are all multitudes. Whether because of the richness of our genetic history or the mind's restless capacity to absorb, we contain the seeds of everything that is. We see a dancer pirouette and know this self is within the realm of possibility. We identify with a starving child in Africa or a nuclear physicist at Harvard and know, but for the quirks of fate, this could be us.

The self that speaks to a mailman is quite different from the self that is a lover, an expert offering advice, or a mother disciplining a child. The self that is angry is different from the self that is gentle or filled with gratitude. If we don't get stuck in discrete selves, we become an ever changing flow of different selves. And to know the new, we gently let go of the old.[1]

Described in this way, the image of a self or even of many selves appears too concrete, too congealed. Instead, it's helpful to talk about the *activity of selfing*. This activity happens in every single moment as we shift from one encounter with life to another. Letting go of the noun and using the verb, we move from having a self (or selves) to being continuously selfing.[2]

But that's not where most of us are. We have congealed selves or, in the language of Mindfulness Meditation, congealed minds: the mind that plans, the mind that lives in memory, the mind that conjures up fantasies, and last, the mind that judges. The minds think differently, and they're not necessarily in sync with one another. Laura's judging mind was critical of her planning mind. And the mind that dreamed up her fantasies had little to do with the mind that planned for the next day—which, to the dreamer, was totally irrelevant.

The more Laura conjured up a woman lover, the more her judging mind found fault. So she created her fantasies in secret and with the disgrace that only a judging mind can impose. This internal conflict absorbed enough energy to mute much of the rest of her psyche. It was like having some kind of push-me-pull-you creature take up residence within her.

In therapy, Laura learned how to listen with awareness, or to be mindful, of her judging mind. She heard the long harangue of so-called faults it spewed about the way she talked, dressed, or thought about sex. And she insightfully realized this judging mind spoke as if it knew the whole truth, even though the comments were often too extreme, too harsh. Besides, it was tyrannical, which was tiresome. Nevertheless, the harangue continued.

During one session, as she began to tell me about a fantasy, her face became hot and red. I asked her to close her eyes and let herself feel the heat on her face. She was feeling the bodily discomfort that's associated with shame. Soon she reported that she felt as if her entire body were getting smaller, shrinking in an effort to hide. That's when she understood that it was shame that she felt, and it kept her apart from others. It interfered with being close. She needed time to let the mind wander through this insight.

There's an old tale about the Sufi seer Nasruddin, who was wandering the streets at four A.M. early one morning when a policeman approached him and asked, "Why are you out wandering in the middle of the night?"

"Sir," replied Nasruddin, "if I knew the answer to that question, I would have been home hours ago!"

And so Laura continued to wander through her eroticism as well as her shame. She cradled her so-called defect like a baby, even though it constricted her relationships and diminished her self-respect. Once she was on the path toward healing, however, she became aware of her trouble. So she had no choice but to listen to the conflict between her eroticism and her shame, and to wander as she waited for still other insights.

Then her daughter, Jeanie, came to visit and brought along her lover. Laura watched them care for each other openly, lovingly, with pride. It was enough to boggle her mind. As she tried to let in that information, her shame became glaringly apparent, and she understood that this shame was the mortar that kept her wall of distraction so thick. And most remarkably, because it stood between her and her daughter, she was determined to take the wall down.

That's when Laura began to talk more openly about her fantasies. This was both relieving and frightening to her; she knew that secrecy protected her from the judging minds of others, and there wasn't any way to stop all those others in the world who are homophobic. The very best I could offer was an affirmation of her strength along with some coaching on how, when necessary, to brace herself against the judging minds of others. All the while, she told her story.

Surprisingly, we realized her parents had eased the way toward a greater self-acceptance by inadvertently modeling their own unconventional sex. The memory of her mother calling *Julia, Julia* in the midst of lovemaking had been a puzzle for Laura for a long time. Retelling the story in therapy, she understood that her mother also felt a passion for women—and somehow she and her father had made it part of their marriage.

Finally, Julia herself helped out with the long forgotten words *You're a jewel, Laura. Trust in that and let yourself shine.* Those words rang out across the years as a gift Laura could finally accept. They opened the door to a new Laura, a woman who could like herself and so accept the is-ness of her sexual orientation. In truth, she was heterosexual *and* homosexual. With the help of Julia and Jeanie she finally accepted her passion for women. Then, quite impressively, she found a way to express that eroticism right in the middle of her marriage. Telling Ned about her fantasy was nothing short of a transformation. It even felt good the next morning.

Mindfulness therapy helped Laura in several ways. She found the courage to name and accept what she thought was her trouble (a sexual interest in women). And it also helped her name the emotions that accompanied her trouble: eroticism and shame.

Recall that emotions are composed of feelings in the body and thoughts in the mind. So, Laura's eroticism was composed of sexual thoughts about women and sexual feelings in her body. She explored both.

The meditation that follows is a tool Laura used to observe the thoughts in her mind. Her challenge was to observe them with the matter-of-factness we call equanimity. This meant listening without judgment. Equanimity is an indispensable state of mind. It's the capacity to stand behind the self and, at the same time, watch the self. Ultimately, equanimity gave Laura the power to break out of the mental prison of shame.

Once again, we'll start with the first meditation on Finding the Stillness. It's a concentration meditation, helpful in calming the mind. Then we'll move on to the object of this chapter's meditation: the thinking mind.

In the previous two meditations, the object of awareness has been the body, both the more physiologically determined sensations we called *external touch* and the more emotionally determined sensations we called *internal feel*. Now your attention will be on the nature of thought. To identify the thinking mind, simply say your name out loud. Then repeat it silently to yourself. The latter is your thinking mind or, as we call it, *internal talk*.

Most people hear their internal talk somewhere between the ears and toward the back of their head, although you may experience it at a different location. Take the time to discover the place of internal talk in your own body. If you can't pinpoint it, simply place your awareness inside your two ear canals. Then rest your awareness there and listen inwardly to your internal talk.[3]

You might hear clear words, so clear that you can repeat them. You might hear a subtle suggestion of talk but nothing that makes sense. Alternatively, you might hear nothing. Any one of the three is fine. The object of this part of the meditation is to keep contact with the place where internal talk takes place. This is not easy to do, because, as a beginner, you're likely to get lost in your internal talk. If so, just return to your two ears and clarify whether what you hear is clear, subtle, or completely absent.

In a third phase of this meditation, you'll have the experience of analyzing thought. Remember, your internal talk might produce *fantasy*, during which you might think of yourself as a queen or a bag lady. It can be a source of deep pleasure and creativity and, as in Laura's case, a means of escape.

You might, instead, find yourself *planning* for what might happen next year or making a list of things that have to happen later on today. The workaholic does this to her detriment; the scientist might use that same capacity to design an experiment that benefits us all. Laura used it to produce films.

Internal talk can also stretch into the past, plowing for memories to tie together events and create a sense of coherence in life. This activity we can call *memory*. While doing this, Laura finally received the gift Julia had given her a long time ago: *You're a jewel, Laura. Trust in that and let yourself shine.*

Last, internal talk can give value to experience. Used skillfully, this *judging mind* has led to outstanding examples of ethical thinking; used unskillfully, it has led to the atomic bomb. Laura struggled mightily with her judging mind. For a long time it berated her for her homosexual thoughts; they were judged to be wrong. That thought pattern led her to hide from everyone, including her family. When she explored this in psychotherapy and became mindful of her judging mind in meditation, the thought pattern lost some of its energy.

During the meditation that follows you'll watch your mind *planning, judging, in memory,* or *in fantasy.* Becoming aware of what internal talk you favor and what you ignore leads to a greater understanding of yourself. But remember, the meditative approach suggests that you not try to make things different in your mind, that you not force yourself to change. However, listening closely might lead to the insight that you don't have to be imprisoned in any of these minds.

Now settle into a chair or a cushion. Use the CD, if you like. And don't forget your timer. If you decide to use the written instructions, read the whole piece first, then return to the first section to follow the instructions. Then meditate, trusting in the wellspring of creativity that lies within you. After all, you, too, are a manifestation of the larger whole.

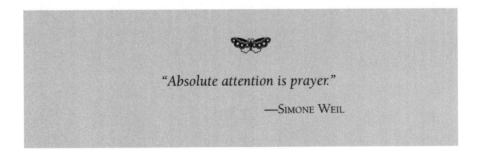

"Absolute attention is prayer."

—Simone Weil

A Meditation on the Thinking Mind

Close your eyes and settle into the body. Allow your shoulders to drop an inch or two . . . and your stomach to loosen. Please repeat the chapter 1 meditation called "A Meditation on Finding the Stillness." Take five minutes to calm the mind.

❧

When you're ready, make the object of this meditation your two ear canals. Then say your name out loud . . . and repeat it silently, to yourself. The latter is **internal talk.**

Now continue to listen. You may not catch the talk as it happens . . . but just a little later . . . after it fades. That's fine.

What you hear may make sense and be **clear** *enough for you to repeat. If so, label that* clear.

What you hear may be subtle . . . just bits and pieces of words that make no sense. If so, label that subtle.

Alternatively, you may hear no thought at all. That's all right. Just label it none.

There's no right or wrong way to do this meditation . . . it's okay to be late . . . it's okay to miss a comment . . . it's okay to guess what you missed . . . or to space out. Just gently bring yourself back to the object of meditation . . . your two ear canals . . . and listen for **internal talk.**

Simply note "clear," "subtle," or "none" and wait for the next talk to arise.

You may realize that the moment you focus on internal talk . . . it disappears. That happens . . . just wait for a few moments and it will return.

You may respond to this difficult meditation by getting sleepy. If so . . . open your eyes . . . and straighten your spine . . . and return to the object of meditation . . . your two ear canals and internal talk . . .

Be gentle with yourself.

Set your timer for five minutes and continue this meditation.

❧

When this time is over . . . continue to keep your awareness at your ear canals . . . continue to listen for internal talk . . . but this time, label what you hear with one of the four categories planning . . . judging . . . memory . . . or fantasy.

If a thought doesn't quite fit . . . forget about it and go on to the next thought. If an external sound captures your attention . . . gently turn back to the place where you hear internal conversation. And wait.

If a body sensation such as an itch on your nose or a pain in your back arises, allow for the sensation . . . and gently return to the place where you hear internal talk . . . be curious and maintain your equanimity.

If no thought arises . . . that's also fine. Label it none *and enjoy the peace.*

Set your timer for ten minutes and continue this meditation.

❀

Now . . . let go of that. This time, keep your awareness at your two ears . . . and name the trouble you've been working with in the previous meditations.

Keeping that trouble in mind . . . listen. You may find yourself in a fantasy . . . in your judging mind . . . remembering the past . . . or planning for the future. Label the category.

Does any of the internal talk have to do with your trouble? Is it totally unrelated? Stay aware . . . everything is information.

And if no thought arises . . . that's okay . . . just enjoy the peace.

Set your timer for five minutes and continue this part of the meditation.

❀

Now slowly open your eyes . . . and sit in the quiet for a few minutes.

If possible, continue to explore the mind in your daily life. Whether at lunch or while waiting in line, take a moment to be aware of the mind, especially if it is focused on your trouble, and label your thoughts . . . fantasy, judging, memory, or planning. Learn about your preferred way of thinking.

It's particularly challenging to meditate on internal talk. So take a moment to compliment yourself for trying. You have done something important.

May all beings know mental happiness.

Training for Awareness

1. Repeat "A Meditation on Finding the Stillness."

2. Keep contact with the ear canals. Listen for internal talk. Label *clear, subtle,* or *none.*

3. Keep contact with the ear canals. Listen for internal talk. Label *planning, judging, memory,* or *fantasy.*

4. Keep contact with the ear canals. Recall the trouble you're working with. Label *planning, judging, memory,* or *fantasy.*

Four

Maria

I suppose I shouldn't be telling you this story. It's really too private. And my family would be horrified if they knew I told. But one of the most important things I've learned in this life is that truth-telling is healing, at least for me. So please don't judge me too harshly when you hear what I have to say. I do enough of that myself.

Steve left me one evening after I refused to have sex with him. It wasn't the first time. He said it wasn't because he didn't love me or anything like that, it was just that he couldn't take it anymore. For the life of me I couldn't blame him. People called me beautiful. Women were jealous of my olive skin and my pale green eyes; they murmured that my figure was sexy, but behind my back they said I was a tramp. I was.

The farewell scene took place in our South Philadelphia row house, right near the Italian market and close to the church where we were both baptized. Many of our relatives and friends lived nearby. We bought the house when Steve got his first full-time job as an electrician. I was already the head of an accounts payable department in a small drug company. We used my savings to make the down payment, and he agreed to take care of the ongoing expenses. Once we got married, it would be our home.

Steve and his brother were remodeling the house after work. When we broke up, they were in the middle of installing new plumbing and heating systems, so the bedroom was just a place to crash, with peeling paint, no curtains, and furniture that was dumped wherever it happened to land. But the bed was ours to use as we could. Of course, I couldn't stay overnight until we were official.

"There's something wrong, Maria," Steve said, sitting bolt upright in the bed. "It's over a week since we had sex, and you still aren't interested. And before that, almost a month went by. I know you're going to say you're upset about work today, but you're always upset," he added cynically, "or tired or sick or worried."

"I wish you would believe me," I answered angrily. "It really *was* a hard day. The accounts payable columns didn't balance out, and my boss got angry. I worked for hours trying to get them straight, but I just couldn't find the error. So when I got into bed with you this evening it was to rest, that's all. I even told you so!"

Steve's face got red. "You're not too tired to go out with your friends until one or two in the morning. You even get up early to get to work. How come you're too tired when it comes to me? For all I know, you're running around with someone else. It happened in the past; why shouldn't it happen now?"

I hesitated, not wanting to hurt him any more than I already had, but the truth was, when he touched me, I felt slightly nauseous. Steve certainly wasn't the most attractive man I had ever dated; he had quite a paunch for a twenty-seven-year-old. But he was kind and gentle, and he loved me like no one else ever had. How could I do this to him?

"I'm telling you straight, Maria. I want to marry you, but not the way you are. Whatever's bothering you, you've got to get over it. Your problems are driving me crazy. God knows I've tried to make this relationship work. Right from the beginning I tried. Remember how I used to protect you whenever you got into trouble in high school? And you got into trouble a lot. Not that I'm complaining. I liked taking care of you. When we got serious after high school, I was so happy I could barely keep my feet on the ground. I've always loved you," he added with a sigh, "and I always will. But I won't get married the way things are."

I could see Steve was getting ready to recite our entire story once again. I wanted to die each time he did it. The mess we were in was my fault; there was no denying it. I was to blame.

"I didn't have any doubts about us the first time we tried to get married, Maria. I knew we were right for each other. And when you had an automobile accident the day before the wedding, I thought it was just bad luck. So I sat down at the telephone and called all one hundred and fifty people to tell them not to come."

"We *both* wanted to get married, Steve, not just you. The accident wasn't my fault. A car swerved out of its lane on the turnpike and hit me. I spent my wedding day in a hospital bed with some broken ribs. It was no fun!"

He held his head and sighed. "I don't know what's true anymore. But it really doesn't matter. Six months ago when we tried again, you got sick a week before. I know the doctor thought you might have muscular dystrophy, and of course I was relieved when he turned out to be wrong, but the fact is, you avoided getting married once again. Fortunately, that time I had to apologize to only fifty people.

"I must have been crazy to want to try again. Here we are, with still another wedding date only two months away, and I know it won't happen. Now it's clear even to me that you don't want to get married. When we first started to go out you were freer," he said, "so much more sensual. You're a different person now. You've got to find out what's wrong!"

I listened to the sound of a lone car speeding down the street in front the house and wished I were in it. But I wasn't, so I avoided his last words and finally whispered, "You're right Steve. With all the trouble we have, we can't get married. I'm afraid something even more terrible will happen if we do. This isn't right. You deserve someone better, someone who can love you the way you want to be loved. I'm trouble for you, Steve, just plain trouble."

That's when he got out of bed, pulled on some clothes, and spit out his decision. "That's just fine with me, Maria. I've had enough too. I'm glad you were the one who said it first. I'm finished, done."

Walking out of the bedroom, he added, "I'm going over to see my Dad. Be gone by the time I return, and take your clothes with you."

I sobbed into the pillow for what seemed like an eternity. How awful I was, how unworthy of this man. Though Steve didn't know for sure, he was sensing there was another man in the picture. Unfortunately, he was right. Oh God, how could I have done this to him? It was just a fling. The guy was twelve years older than I, married, and not the kind who leaves his wife. Even though we were drawn to each other like two powerful magnets, I knew it could end at any moment. Crazy as it sounds, I could have sex with a guy who didn't care about me; but I couldn't have sex with the man I was supposed to marry.

Why did God make me so pretty if I couldn't handle it? At my worst I thought it was a test I had already failed. I was a sinner, rotten to the core. Even my name was a problem. How could I ever live up to Mary, mother of Christ, the Madonna? Don't misunderstand me; it's not that I didn't try to be good. I certainly worried about it enough. But no matter how baggy my clothes and how light my makeup, men came on to me. I was a piece of candy they could easily gobble up. After all, candy can't resist.

So Steve and I stopped seeing each other. Well, that's not exactly right—actually we stopped trying to be lovers, but that old friendship of ours continued to limp along. My relationship with the married guy also ended. It had to. I desperately wanted to be good, so I vowed to stay away from men. Each morning on the way to work, I went to church and prayed to God for help. Each evening I rushed home and sat in front of the television. But it wasn't long before I slipped again.

My boss took me and six others to San Francisco on a business trip. Drinking too much was the first mistake. But it got worse. When the alcohol wore off, it was two in the morning and I was sitting in my boss's lap right in the middle of the hotel lobby. The next day the women from the office avoided my eyes and the men were a little too familiar.

Can you understand how horrible that failure was for me? For years I had been feeling that there was something separating me from others. I called it my glass bubble. From the outside I probably looked cool and disinterested. Inside, I felt terribly self-conscious and frightened, sure that others hated me as much as I hated myself. After this failure, the bubble got even thicker, and I felt hopeless. Whatever made me a tramp, it couldn't be stopped. I thought of leaving town. I even thought of killing myself. But instead I continued to live the way I always had, only things got worse. Guys came in and out of my life and I drank more than ever to drown my shame. Relatives and friends began passing me by in the street. It didn't matter. I really didn't want to talk to them. Only Steve stayed in touch, but barely. I felt too guilty to let him in.

So life went, until one day, having lunch with a friend in our local greasy spoon, a bulb clicked on in my head. My friend confided that she was a survivor of incest. At first I thought her story had nothing to do with me, but I was spellbound and asked many more questions than I should have. And then I knew it had everything to do with me.

"I think my father had sex with me when I was fifteen," I confessed. "It hasn't ever been a big deal, maybe because it happened only once, and no one ever talked about it. Besides, the memory isn't clear, and sometimes I believe it's only my imagination."

"Even the possibility that incest happened is important," she explained. "Why shouldn't it be?"

And so I went to the next meeting of my friend's incest survivors group, which happened to take place in my very own church. Going turned out to be one of the best things I ever did. Much to my amazement, the women didn't seem to be ashamed of themselves. And many of their stories were much worse than mine! All I could do was cry, and please understand, I'm not a person who cries easily, especially in front of other people. Even more remarkably, for the first time in my life I began to ask out loud the questions that had haunted me for years.

Why, I wondered, had my mother insisted that I spend time alone with Dad even though I tried to refuse? How come she slapped my face when I told her what had happened between Dad and me? And why, when I asked her recently, couldn't my sister talk to me about her memories of Dad? Simply getting the questions out made me feel less like a sinner. Maybe, if I found the answers, my glass bubble would burst and I'd be able to get on with my life.

So I found myself a therapist, and sure enough over the next year things began to change, including my naive belief that the next frog who offered love would turn into a prince. I think this happened because I started to look inside for my answers. I talked and talked in therapy—and in my group—about my father's behavior. And slowly, remarkably, I quit blaming myself for it. It helped to meditate on the voice inside that judged me so mercilessly. Not that the voice ever went away, but after a while it didn't have quite the same power. Then it seemed to be an easier step to accept the reality that I really was sexually abused.

Even as I tell you this, I'm amazed at how hard that acceptance was. I even considered the idea that I was a woman of great courage. After all, I had managed to keep my sanity. I was a survivor!

But there was a challenge I had to face. The women in my incest survivors group believed that confronting the person who had sexually abused them was an important step toward healing. Some of them had done this. We all felt tremendously proud when one of us could hold her own in front of her abuser, although as far as I knew not one of their fathers ever admitted to the abuse. Nevertheless, I decided to try it myself, in hope that the ordeal would set me free.

I was fairly sure my father wouldn't be willing to go to a therapy session with me; frankly, even the thought triggered that old seething anger in the pit of my stomach. I hated the man. Anyway, I had no way of reaching him. He left our family about the time I went away to college and had been wandering back and forth across the country ever since. Once in a long while he would show up, but no one could predict when. The only thing I could do was wait. Sure enough, after several months, he finally appeared at my front door.

He looked awfully sick—in his head as well as in his body. I made him dinner and listened to the long, depressing story of his lonely trip across the country. Ugh, it was awful to hear. Finally, I screwed up my courage and launched in: "Dad, I have something important to ask you. I'm seeing a therapist and she wants you to come to a session. Would you go with me?"

I guess he was so thankful I had taken him in that he couldn't say no. And, of course, I didn't even hint at what I really wanted to talk about. That would have gotten him angry.

And so it happened that early one summer evening my father and I walked into my therapist's office. Dad looked disheveled and a little confused. I was all business in my dark blue suit with my hair swept up, ready to be competent and tough. In truth, I was terrified.

After the introductions, I launched in quickly, probably too quickly, and then I couldn't stop. "I remember when I first found out you were having sex with my little sister, Dad. It was on my thirteenth birthday. I was looking for one of my presents in Abby's bedroom and instead spotted an envelope poking out from under her pillow. It was in your handwriting. I felt guilty opening it, but I did anyway. You sent her a picture of a big red heart with lace around it, and underneath you wrote, 'A heart for my pretty daughter.' It wasn't her birthday, it was mine. So I asked Abby about the note, thinking maybe it was a mistake. She told me the whole truth, Dad, the whole truth. She was only eleven at the time."

Halfway through my speech I heard myself sounding like a whining child. I even started to cry. Gone was the tough woman I had wanted to be. There was nothing to do but go on anyway. "I felt devastated by that note, Dad, not because of the incest, I didn't even know the word, but because you were more interested in Abby than me. Crazy as it sounds, I thought there was something wrong with me because I wasn't the chosen one. I was such a skinny little thing and my acne was awful."

My father sat directly across from me, bent over, with his arms wrapped tightly around his chest, looking down at his shoes. I expected him to yell and scream at me, but that didn't happen. So I continued. "I *hated* you and Abby, and I hated all that secrecy. I was left out in the cold. It was cruel! I wanted you to pay attention to *me*, to put *me* on your lap, not Abby. Insane, isn't it, to hold on to such a hopeless dream?

"Worse still, you were almost always irritated with me, if not downright angry, especially after you had a few drinks. I can't tell you how many times you told me I was my mother's child, too timid to be a child of yours. Meanwhile, Mom seemed to be in a world of her own."

Pausing, I hoped my father would say something or even just move a muscle. But he didn't. Looking back seemed to have turned him into a pillar of salt. The silence in the office roared in my ears, as if the crimson velvet couch and the soft gray chairs were determined to wait it out and hear the truth. Even the children playing in the street grew quiet.

I went on. "Almost everything in our family life got confused with sex. Remember how you loved being nude? Every morning we girls would watch you admire yourself in the mirror before you put on your clothes. Every day we had to put up with your affection: 'I deserve some real kisses from my gals before I leave the house,'" I mimicked. "And as soon as you came home at night you would take off all your clothes again. I can't tell you how much I wished you would love me like a normal dad, with a smile, a pat on the back, or even some help with my homework. But that's not the way it turned out.

"Now, here's where my memory becomes vague. I think I was fifteen when, for some reason I can't remember, Mom and Abby went away and the two of us were alone for a day and a night in that house. I recall being very nervous and trying to avoid you. Over dinner, I think you talked about the tension between us, which made me even more nervous. You said closeness would help, that we could make it better if I let you hold me. So after dessert you took my hand and led me to your bed. I laid down, shivering. Then I have a vivid image of you walking toward me from the bathroom door, without any clothes on and your penis erect. 'I'm all yours,' you said. 'I'm all yours.'"

"No, no," my father roared, finally breaking his silence. "I wasn't the one who wanted sex. It was you! Admit it, you were the one who asked for it, not me. I wasn't really attracted to you. I did it for us. That's the honest truth!"

Sobbing, I swallowed hard and continued. "Almost as soon as it was over, I felt terribly ashamed. How could I have let myself do this? Why did I listen to you? I stood under the shower for what seemed like hours washing and washing, trying to get off all the filth. Worse, the very next day the truth became clear even to me; having sex didn't change anything. You still loved Abby more than you loved me."

His gray eyes flat, my father tried to justify himself. "I know you want me to say that we had sex. And I'll do that for you, Maria. I do admit that sex took place. That's true. But try to understand, there's nothing wrong with sex. Society makes it wrong. Otherwise, sex is just a way to be close. Don't you realize that when we got together that night it was because I loved you?"

"How can you say that?" I yelled. "It's *wrong* for a father and a daughter to have sex! Don't you know that? What's the matter with you? For years I've blamed myself for having sex with you. As long as I can remember I've felt guilty about it. And now, just when I've begun to doubt I'm a whore, you tell me it's my fault? Finally I understand that what I wanted all these years was a just little love—not sex."

"Please help me," I pleaded. "Don't make me the bad one again, Dad."

Sitting back in his chair, my father folded his arms back across his chest and declared, "You were the one who wanted it. Don't deny it. You know I wasn't attracted to you."

That got me even more angry. "You never think about me. How can you say something so mean and rejecting! And what happened to the old-fashioned idea that a father should protect his daughter? Doesn't that mean anything to you? This is wrong, Dad. How can a father blame his fifteen-year-old daughter for taking part in incest?"

We walked out of the office angrily that day, avoiding even a glance at each other. And I expected to be up most of the night reliving the horror of my early years. When my therapist called the next morning to ask how I was, I told her it really was a hard night, but I woke up feeling proud of myself. "Did you notice?" I asked. "There wasn't any glass bubble around me. I wasn't hiding. Besides, now I know for sure my memory is real; my father did have sex with me."

"By the way," I added, "he left town just a few hours ago. He put on a real performance last night. It took hours. At one point, he even threatened to kill himself. Frankly, I don't care. This time around I want him to know he's not the only one who's important."

A full year passed before my father returned. He looked even more disheveled than I remembered, but not so confused. This didn't surprise me—often he could sound fairly rational—even when what he said really didn't make sense. I asked if he would go to another therapy session with me. Surprisingly, he seemed to want to come.

We drove to that session in silence. I was afraid to be hopeful.

"I've decided to tell you the truth about what happened to me during this past year," he began. "You may still end up hating me, but I have to take that chance. I spent most of this past year alone trying not to think about killing myself. I was lonelier than I've ever been in my life. No one to talk to. No one to love. I was desperate."

It's the same old stuff, I thought to myself. The same old "poor me, poor me." I can't stand it anymore!

Meanwhile he continued, "One night, in a movie theater in Kansas City, I had a tremendous urge to touch the thigh of the little girl sitting next to me. She was sitting so close that I could feel the heat of her body. Her bare leg was only inches away. You have no idea how torturous it was. Somehow I had to know if I was still alive, and I was sure the touch of her skin would do it. I struggled against the urge for most of the movie, but finally let the back of my hand rub down her leg. What happened next was awful; I wanted to die. The girl screamed and her mother accused me in front of all those people in the theater. The police finally came and hauled me into jail. I was released only when I agreed to go to a therapy group for men like me."

"Why can't people understand me?" he pleaded. "What happened didn't mean anything. I wasn't going to hurt her. The judge actually had the nerve to say I was a dangerous and destructive person. What's the matter with him? This is all absurd. Touching isn't bad. Why don't they know that?

"I attended those group therapy meetings for a while, but they weren't for me. I could see that. Everyone kept asking me to apologize for what I did. But how could I do that when I really didn't believe I did anything wrong? So I finally gave up, packed my bags, and came home to Philadelphia."

Taking a crumpled letter out of his pocket, he explained, "The therapist tracked me down and sent this letter just a few days ago. I'd like to read it aloud so you both can see how badly I was treated, how little they understood me.

Dear William,

I urge you to come back to Kansas and attend our group sessions. We all care about you, although we won't tolerate the excuses you use to justify your sexual assaults on young girls. We believe you simply have no idea what it means to a girl when you touch her in ways that intrude on her privacy. It's intolerable.

I repeat, we are concerned for you, but we cannot take part in the cover-up, the excuses, the conspiracy of silence that has allowed you to sexually abuse children for so much of your life. It's just plain wrong and has damaged you as well as others.

Please call,

Steve

My father put down the letter and continued without a pause. "In my opinion, all these men have father issues, and I'm a convenient target. That's exactly what I said to the therapist and the men in my group, but they got angry and kept demanding that I talk about what they called my 'inappropriate' sex life . . . "

"*Dad, stop!*" I interrupted. "*Stop* using the same old excuses, all the crazy ideas, the garbage that I've heard all of my life. I don't want it anymore. I can't stand it. Forget about yourself. Forget about Kansas City even. Just think about me, think about what you did to your daughter! Why did you have sex with me? Why couldn't you do it with your wife or people your own age? Don't you know having it with your daughter is bad? Why can't you understand that I wanted affection, not sex? And I know Abby did too. How could you even think of having sex with your own children?

"I want to hear that you know you did wrong, and that you mean it. I need to hear those words over and over again until they sink in, until I can count on them."

My father didn't change his story. "I'm sorry it happened, Maria, but you wanted it. I kept thinking that if we went through it together, sex would help solve the problem between us. That's why I went along with you."

We left the office very angry at each other.

Several weeks later, he called me and suggested still another session with my therapist. He sounded serious and maybe even a little clearheaded, so I said okay. Could it be that confronting him in front of my therapist was making a difference? Or was this just another ploy to get me to take care of him? Whichever, I was determined that this meeting was his last chance, at least with me.

"Please hear me," he began tearfully, with more honest feeling than I had ever heard from him. "I am sorry. It was wrong to have sex with you. I am your father and I shouldn't have put you through this. It's no excuse, but I didn't think it would hurt you. I didn't know."

"How come you've changed, Dad? I don't know if I can trust you," I responded, rather cynically. "I know you. You'll try anything to be accepted."

"Please let me try to convince you. You're the only one I can turn to. Your mother won't have me. Your sister won't speak to me. I want to try to tell you I'm sorry."

"Okay, Dad, I'll listen. But don't expect anything from me in return. I can't make your life better. I don't even want to."

"If only I could undo the harm I did," he continued. "I want to be a better father to you. I really do. I've never told you before, but I was also abused by my father. It wasn't sexual; he did it through beatings. I tried to keep it private so you would think well of your grandfather, but now I know that was wrong. Every Saturday night, he would come home drunk and find some excuse to beat me. In comparison with him, I thought I was being a good father, that I was loving you, not beating you. I'm really sorry I hurt you like he hurt me, and I would do anything in the world to change what happened. But it did happen. I couldn't love you like a father should."

Despite my anger at him, tears streamed down my face, and I said, "Thank you, Dad, thank you. I hope you can find the love you want with someone more fitting."

And after a few moments of silence, I added, "But please hear me, right now I can't offer you more than that. Strange, I've dreamed of this moment for so long, and I always thought I would instantly forgive you. But that's not what I feel. I can't really believe that you feel sorry. I just can't trust you. I wish it could be different, but I can't find that forgiveness in my heart."

My father cried and said nothing.

Over the next months, I did try to forgive him, but I knew that I had to find that forgiveness in my heart, and whenever I tried, I found nothing but numbness. I just couldn't trust him. Blaming myself didn't help either. It just didn't happen.

My father did give me an important gift, but I still couldn't stand to be with him. I decided not to welcome him into my house any longer. I would help him with money if he was in trouble, and I would talk to him over the telephone, but I wouldn't see him. I just didn't want to.

Steve and I had been just friends for several years by that time. We went everywhere together, the beach, good restaurants, the movies. People couldn't understand our relationship. Some even thought it was wrong. But that didn't matter; we cared about each other.

Maybe it was because I felt better that we began to do better. My old self-consciousness was mostly gone, and with every week that passed I seemed to feel easier with people. I was even learning how to manage the men who came on to me. Finally, after all these years, I realized I could enjoy their attention and still not do what they asked. Walking down that old road wasn't going to give me what I wanted. I knew it in my bones.

And then I began to think of Steve as a man. I realized it was a true feeling because my skin tingled whenever I had the thought. A miracle was happening, and I wasn't going to doubt it. Instead, I invited him out to dinner and, in a quiet moment, confided that I really did love him. I even said I wanted us to make a baby together. When he said he could think of nothing better than to make a baby with me, I was ecstatic! Since then my life has changed.

Not that we're without troubles. When I went away on a business trip a while ago, Steve called every day to ask who I was with, what I was doing, and why. I knew he was worried that I might go off with someone else, even though I told him I wouldn't.

As you can probably guess, Steve and I finally did get married, but only after we knew I was pregnant. The church ceremony was small, with just the two of us, my sister with her family, and his parents. I had no problem getting to that wedding. And I loved being pregnant. It was one of the most joyful times in my life.

Meanwhile, my father stopped wandering around the country, rented an apartment in Baltimore, and got a job. More important, he found a new woman friend who was only ten years younger than he.

Every morning I go to church and thank God for what has happened. Now I can say for sure I'm not a tramp. And I'm not walking around in that glass bubble anymore. Instead, I'm the proud mother of a beautiful baby girl who is also named Maria. Steve and I want to raise her to be proud of that name. She will be baptized tomorrow.

"As we let our own light shine, we unconsciously give other people the freedom to do the same. As we are liberated from our own fear our presence automatically liberates others."

—MAYA ANGELOU

HEAVEN AND HELL

Here's an old tale about heaven and hell. Perhaps it will shed some light on Maria's complex and difficult story.

One day a big, brawny samurai came to visit a Zen master and asked, "Please tell me about the nature of heaven and hell."

This Zen master sat quietly for a while and then responded angrily: "Why should I tell a dirty, repulsive, wretched man like you such important information? Who are you to even ask?"

Furious, the samurai got red in the face and screamed and cursed. This didn't stop the Zen master from continuing, "What a disgusting miserable snake you are. Look at yourself; you're despicable. Why do you, of all people, think I should tell you anything?"

Consumed with rage, the samurai drew his sword and was about to behead the Zen master when, just in time, the wise man bellowed, "That's hell."

The samurai instantly understood the teaching. Tears filled his eyes as he put his palms together to bow.

"That's heaven," concluded the Zen master.

Heaven and hell are right here on earth. People create them by the way they think. Hell can be a self-absorption so total there's almost no room for the humanity of anyone else. For example, Maria's father could see no further than the pain of his loneliness. For him, little girls had no feelings; they were simply things to use. Besides, they didn't have much capacity to say no, which made them excellent prey.

Maria created her own hell inside her glass bubble. She, too, was immersed in pain. Not that she could identify its causes—the fog of confusion and desolation was too dense. And she, too, was caught in an effort to break out through sex. They were disconnected, unfeeling attempts to relieve her loneliness. Of course, the men *she* used had a capacity to protect themselves, so her behavior was many degrees less horrendous than her father's use of little girls. But she was isolated, guilty, and filled with self-hatred.

I recall sitting with Maria the first time she came to see me. She was truly a beautiful woman, but her features were stiff, frozen. She rarely smiled, and the small muscles around the eyes that facilitate expression seemed not to work. It was hard to relate to her. Trying to empathize, I seemed to run up against her glass bubble. Nor was it easy to relate to her father; he was preoccupied with his disorganized thoughts.

Both Maria and her father suffered from the trauma of abuse. Being exploited and mistreated early in life, they sensed that something terrible was wrong with them and believed they were corrupt, sinful outcasts. To the rest of the world, however, beautiful Maria presented herself as perfection incarnate. And her father, with all his capacity to charm people through words, presented himself as intelligent, even insightful. Maintaining these facades was hard work; it absorbed them, devouring much of their psychic energy. In fact, they were caught in that hell of a self-absorption so total that it isolated them from others.

This is the psychological problem called *narcissism*. The word derives from the Greek myth about a beautiful young boy named Narcissus who fell in love with his own image in a pool of still water along the river's edge. It was the most beautiful image he had ever seen. However, when he touched the face in the water, which he supposed was a water nymph, it trembled and disappeared. He was so in love and, I might add, so desperately lonely that he vowed to continue looking at the nymph until it appeared in the flesh and loved him. Eventually his legs grew into the bank of the river to become roots, his hair grew long and leafy, and his face became the beautiful flower called the narcissus.[1]

At one and the same time, Narcissus was in search of himself and captured by his own reflection. Indeed, he ultimately became the reflection and so lost his human form. Many contemporary psychotherapists, particularly Donald W. Winnicott and Heinz Kohut, interpret the story to mean that Narcissus was captured by the dream of perfection. This dream ultimately became a false self that hid, and actually destroyed, his humanly flawed, true self.

Narcissism is associated with symptoms that come along with this false self. Narcissists have a lack of empathy, an undying need for admiration, a sense of emptiness that leads them to believe they're frauds, and the experience of isolation. These symptoms appear whether they idealize themselves or depreciate themselves. In both cases, those who are afflicted hurt so much that they're preoccupied with themselves.[2]

Buddhists understand this differently than psychotherapists do. They understand this person to be caught in the effort to find the self, which is a problem because the self is nowhere to be found. That's because the self is not a thing but instead a range of mind/body sensations that come and go. Indeed, the more we human beings try to grasp for the self, the more frightened we become. And in that fear, we hold on to the phantom self ever more tightly, ever more rigidly. In effect, we fear our own insubstantiality. But that's like fearing the rising and setting of the sun. It just is.[3]

Compared to the suffering that self-absorption caused in the lives of Maria and her father, Narcissus was lucky to have emerged in the form of a beautiful flower. The samurai didn't fare so well either; self-absorption led him to behave like a killer, although he ultimately avoided this fate by means of a great insight into the nature of heaven and hell. Maria and her father also found a way out of their own hell, this time through truth-telling.

At best, truth-telling is an interactive dance that cracks open the preoccupation with self. Doing it is dangerous, particularly if the person who is listening is deeply committed to denying the truth-teller's information. That's when interactions are likely to become hostile. For this

reason, Maria wasn't able to confront her father until she had my support and the support of her incest survivors group.

Of interest to me as a psychotherapist was that by the time Maria,
her father, and I came together to talk about the abuse, she knew exactly
what to do; she had practiced the words in her incest survivors group,
listened to the experience of others who had confronted their abusers,
even practiced the expression of the anger, deep hurt, and the feeling of
empowerment that comes with asserting oneself before an abuser. The
incest survivor movement had taught her well. Without it, I doubt this
story could have been told. Maria, her father, and I were part of an inter-
dependent healing community for victims of abuse that exists in our
country and probably across much of the world—even though we don't
know each other. The power of good in people is truly astounding.

Truth-telling was far from easy for Maria's father. He had to find his
way through confusion, blame, denial, and the kind of self-hatred that
might have ended in suicide. Maria was better prepared, not only because of her incest survivors group but also because she was able to use
the tools of Mindfulness Psychotherapy to work with the emotions that
arose inside her whenever she faced her own truths. Over time, as she
learned to watch her emotions arise, manifest, and fade, their power
lessened. It felt as if she were shedding a skin.

But this wasn't enough to heal the rift between father and daughter.
For that to happen, their truth-telling would have had to be coupled
with loving compassion. This is not the kind of love that overlooks personal responsibility or moves quickly into forgiveness. Instead, it's the
capacity to be with another's pain and offer comfort. Neither Maria nor
her father could do that. Their own pain was too deep, and their suffering too great. And so, after all the talking was over and much of the
blame had dissipated, Maria tried to forgive her father but couldn't. Love
for him was nowhere to be found; she just felt numb. To her credit, she
didn't blame herself or cover her numbness with anger. Instead, she felt
grounded in her truth.

And she felt proud of what she had accomplished. Maria had found
a way to name and accept the *is-ness* of her early abuse, and the emotions it triggered. She had learned to listen to her judging mind with

equanimity, which she likened to being on an airplane and looking down at the tortuous canyons and the beautiful plains of the earth, all the while knowing that neither one was better than the other. They both had their place. Similarly, looking down at herself, she saw a woman who got caught in an abusive drama and now was leaving it.

During one of her therapy sessions, while telling me how she drank too much on a business trip and came to in the wee hours of the morning to find herself sitting on her boss's lap, Maria heard her judging mind call her a whore. I asked her to close her eyes and watch how her ribs expanded on the in-breath and contracted on the out-breath. When I sensed that her body was relaxed, I guided her back to the memory of herself sitting on her boss's lap and asked her to listen to her judging mind. Sure enough, her self-hatred arose again. In a meditative state, she could listen very closely. Many thoughts surfaced, but the phrase "I'm a whore" was very loud and clear. It came with a body sensation she described as "shrinking with shame."

Over time and with equanimity, that shrinking-with-shame feeling lessened. And that made room for a different sense of self: She was a woman who was caught in a multigenerational drama about incest, and a woman who could live up to the reputation of her namesake.

You might ask, "Exactly how do you find the equanimity that's needed to listen to the judging mind without bolting?" One way is to bring mindfulness to everyday life. For instance, the next time you hear yourself say *I did this wrong* or *She's no good*, stop for a moment and pay attention. Ask yourself, How often do I hear those same words? How mean are they? And can I listen in a neutral way, objectively accepting the is-ness of the words?

Another way to explore equanimity is to sit in a busy restaurant, close your eyes, and listen to all the sound around you at once. If you listen without any internal talk, you'll hear the waves of conversation—sound rising and falling all around you like waves in the sea. No one sound is better or worse. You're open to all of it because in your own small way, even through the subtle sound of your breath, you're part of it. Letting go of discrimination can give you a direct sense of the peace that comes with wholeness.

A third way is to listen to your judging mind while meditating until it becomes nothing more than a flow of sound.

Now on to the meditation. As usual, we'll begin with a concentration exercise, and then we'll focus on the thinking mind. While the instruction is simply to listen, as we know, that's not easy to do. But if you're patient you're likely to catch some of your thoughts. Try not to get caught in the content; simply watch the words come and go.

In the third section, the object of the meditation will shift to the judging mind. Make sure to relax into the body repeatedly; the deeper the relaxation, the more open the mind. And when you're ready, create the intention to listen to the judging mind. Of course, it might not emerge. Or it might emerge loudly, in a stream of self-criticism or blame. Whichever, *just listen.* Consider how you relate to your judging mind. Are you surprised to hear what it has to say? Are you upset? Does it blame you or others? Do you think it tells the truth?

In the last part of this meditation you'll explore a method of increasing your equanimity with the judging mind that Shinzen has suggested. By erasing content, it allows you to focus on words as sound. This can lead to the insight that the judging mind is not as powerful as one might believe.

Now it's time to settle on a cushion or a chair. Let's see if the judging mind will expose itself to you; if it does, you'll have the opportunity to become more precise about how it comments on your life—and your trouble. If it doesn't appear, that's all right. Perhaps your mind will settle into planning, memory, or fantasy. Whichever, keep your awareness focused on your ear canals. And remember, anytime you hear yourself think about good or bad, right or wrong, should or shouldn't, you're in the judging mind. (Meanwhile, don't forget your timer and a pad of paper.)

"I am still the place where creation does some work on itself."

—TOMAS TRANSTROMER, TRANSLATED FROM THE SWEDISH BY ROBERT BLY

A Meditation on Equanimity and the Judging Mind

Close your eyes and relax into the body.

Set your timer for five minutes and repeat the meditation called "Finding the Stillness."

❀

When the five minutes are over, place your awareness in the two ear canals, or the place where you hear internal conversation, and listen. It may be hard to catch the thinking mind . . . you may be aware of your internal voice only after it stops speaking . . . or you may hear nothing at all. That's all right. Remember, the object of this section of the meditation is simply to keep contact with the place where you hear internal conversation.

If your awareness shifts to a feeling of discomfort in the body . . . an itch or a pain . . . gently return to your two ears. And label . . . clear . . . subtle . . . none.

Have patience. This is a hard meditation. Just listen.

Set your timer for five minutes and continue meditating.

❀

When the five minutes are over, once again relax into the body. Now, create the intention to be in contact with the judging mind, and listen. You might hear your internal voice blaming others for your trouble. Label that judging.

Maybe . . . instead . . . your judging mind is blaming you. Label that judging.

Or, you might hear nothing at all. If that's true . . . enjoy the peace and label that none. Listen with equanimity to whatever arises.

If outside sounds interfere . . . gently bring your awareness back to your two ear canals and internal talk.

Try not to judge the judging mind. Just listen . . . stay aware . . . accept the fact that the voice exists.

And recall that there's no right way to do this meditation. For some the judging mind will arise . . . for others, it won't.

Set your timer for ten minutes. Let your awareness stay in the place where you hear your internal voice . . . wait and listen. Everything is grist for the mill.

✦

When the ten minutes are over, continue to listen to your internal voice, but this time . . . slow down the voice.

If you hear yourself say, I'm good at this *. . . repeat the phrase so it sounds like* IIIIIImmmm . . . goood . . . . aaat . . . thiiiissss. *Say it so slowly that the meaning is lost and all you hear is sound. Repeat it a few times.*

Begin to recognize that the sound itself is interesting. Watch it arise . . . and fade . . . only to arise again. Let the sound massage the deep recesses of your thinking mind.

Set your timer for five minutes and attend to the sound of your internal talk.

✦

Now place your awareness in your two ear canals and recall the trouble you have been working on. Then listen for judging internal talk.

If your mind wanders, gently return your awareness to your ear canals and listen for your judging mind's comments on your trouble.

If you hear nothing at all . . . just relax.

If you catch your judging mind's comment on your trouble, stretch the words until they're nothing but sound. You did this wrong *might become* youuuuuuuuu diiiiiiiiiiiiiiiiidthiiiiisssswrrrrrronggggggg.

Set your timer for five minutes and keep your awareness at your two ear canals.

✦

When you're ready to end the meditation, simply open your eyes . . . and take a few moments to settle back into everyday life.

You have just experienced mindfulness in action, the capacity to focus your awareness on an aspect of your mind/body process. Indeed, listening with equanimity to what your judging mind has to say may very well lead to one of those insights that shift the way you think about yourself.

You might want to repeat this meditation before you go to sleep or while you're washing the dishes. Do so by placing your awareness in your two ear canals and then listening.

And remember, all beings are manifestations of the larger whole . . . and that is fundamentally good.

May all beings know peace.

Training for Awareness

1. Start with the meditation called "Finding the Stillness."

2. Keep contact with the place where you hear internal talk. Listen and label *clear, subtle,* or *none.*

3. Keep contact with the place where you hear internal talk. Listen for the judging mind. Whatever talk emerges, label *clear, subtle,* or *none.*

4. Keep contact with the place where you hear internal talk. Slow down talk until it becomes nothing but sound.

5. Recall your trouble and listen to your judging mind. Slow down talk until it becomes nothing but sound.

Five

How Nancy Gave Birth
to a Healer

Would you understand what I meant if I told you that the day I lost Max was both the best and the worst day of my life? To know what I had in mind, you might ask me which it really was, and I would have to insist it was both. Then I would explain: the day I lost Max was the day I lost my childhood. In all the years since, I have never felt quite as safe, quite as loved. But if Max had lived, I would never have become a healer.

I wasn't born to be a healer. I was born to be crazy. The way I see it, I've always had the capacity for both. In fact, I tried being crazy for a while when I was a teenager, but it didn't suit. Years later my inner guides pointed me in the right direction . . . but wait a minute, I'm getting ahead of myself. I have to tell you how it all happened.

I was brought up on a farm outside of Uniondale, Pennsylvania, a small town about a hundred and fifty miles northeast of Philadelphia. It wasn't much of a town by the time I came around; all that was left was the post office, a lumberyard, and a grocery with a barber's chair in one of its back rooms. The last time I spoke to the owner of this grocery–barber shop, he told me he and his son had been giving the men of Uniondale haircuts for eighty consecutive years.

In my grandmother's time, Uniondale was a stop on the line between Scranton and Susquehanna, so it also had flaunted a railroad station, a bar, and a hotel. But soon the coal mines closed down, the trains stopped running, and people began to leave. Not so my mother and father. They stayed put.

Our farmhouse was filled with the stuff of several generations. White lace doilies crocheted by my great-grandmother covered the arms of chairs; hand-hooked rugs were spread across the rough pine floors that my great-grandfather laid. My grandmother's picture hung on the wall in the dining room; her dishes showed through the glass of the china cabinet. She lived in that house for fifty years after her oldest child shot and killed herself in the attic. The girl was only fifteen at the time. My grandfather ran away right after, leaving his wife and ten children to fend for themselves. Over the years, all but one, the youngest boy, moved away. That boy farmed the land and eventually married a girl from the next farm over. Soon there were four of us in that house, my grandmother, my mother, my father and I.

Sometimes it's hard for me to believe these are my roots. I would like to think I'm the descendant of a long line of healers; certainly my life would have been easier if that were true. But it's not. My mother and father believed in only what they could touch or see. They were afraid of anything extraordinary.

Max was extraordinary, and that, I think, is why he had to die. I remember as clear as day the moment it happened. I was sitting on the floor of our living room with my favorite doll, Munshka, trying to feed her a special medicine-water I had concocted. Meanwhile my parents were drinking whisky and screaming at each other, about what I did not know. I can even picture my grandmother staring absentmindedly out the window. She never fully recovered from the loss of her daughter and her husband.

As it turned out, Munshka didn't like the taste of the medicine-water and so she spilled it. That upset my mother. "Nancy," she barked, "the water is getting all over the rug." The next thing I knew the big hulk that was my father grabbed me by the arm and tossed me away from the mess.

That's when Max appeared. He always came when I was in trouble. If I had to go to the doctor or if I woke up at night and the room was very dark, Max was sure to help out. Once he even went out with me on Halloween night. This time, he came dressed as a pirate with a patch over his eye. He looked so funny that I laughed.

Suddenly the room became very quiet. "Why are you laughing?" I heard my father ask.

"It's Max. He's dressed funny, like a pirate with a patch over his eye. Don't you see?"

"No," my father responded irritably. "There is no Max. I don't want to hear you say any more about him. You're too old for that kind of play."

My mother agreed, but with a touch of panic in her voice. "Stop it right now, Nancy. There isn't anybody there. It's only your imagination."

"Max is right here," I said, pointing toward him. "Can't you see?"

My father started to pace. He always did that when he was upset. That man knew how to milk cows and cut hay but not how to raise a little girl. If he was angry, all he knew was to use his big hands to push me around. So whenever he began to pace, I got scared. This time Max distracted me.

"Let's play," he said. "You can be a pirate, too. We'll make a boat."

"All right," I answered. "Can we make swords, too?"

The conversation made my father even angrier. Now he was yelling that my mother was making me crazy. "She's going to turn out just like your sister and it's all your fault."

"How can you say it's *my* fault! It's *your* sister who killed herself. It's *your* genes that are the problem. I didn't have anything to do with that."

"But it was *your* sister who spent most of her life in a state institution."

"Yes, but that was because of the accident. She wasn't crazy."

That's when my father stomped into my tiny playground with his huge shoes and tried to grab for Munshka. Somehow he didn't see that Max was sitting a step away from his left foot, so I took a fistful of his pants and pulled hard, but I wasn't strong enough. It was too late.

"*You stepped on Max*" I wailed. "*You killed my best friend.*"

Life was never really the same after that. I was terribly sad and I wasn't supposed to be. According to my parents, Max had to disappear without a tear being shed. But I could no more have stopped that sadness than stop my bones from growing. So I cried alone.

Trouble was, my parents were worried. Not that they ever said anything, but I could sense it. They thought I was "different." And I knew they were watching for signs of my "problem." Once I overheard my mother talking to her friend, saying I was a child with too much "imagination." After this went on for a while, my imagination frightened me as well as my family. I didn't know then that it was a gift I had been granted, a capacity to see what others could not.

When I was fourteen, something happened that convinced me I wasn't normal. Walking in the woods, I looked up at a tree and saw its leaves begin to shudder. That was strange enough, but then I looked around at the other trees and saw there was no movement at all in their leaves. And then I thought I caught a glimpse of a woman in a long white dress far into the woods. What was going on? I wasn't supposed to see things like that. So I panicked and ran as fast as I could out of the woods, back to my house, and hid under the covers of my bed. I never told anyone about it, but that strange sighting confirmed my fear: there was something very wrong with me.

Even so, I was normal enough to learn how to skate. The rink was near Forest City and close to cousin Estelle, which was lucky, because my mother liked to visit her. Skating was fun. I would imagine I was some beautiful bird, maybe a pure white swan with long feathers gliding majestically over the ice. Soon I even had a friend there. She convinced me that I should take lessons with her, and after a few days of begging I managed to get permission from my mother. However, the lessons came with a proviso: no "tricks" on the ice, no jumps, no twirls, no speed. They were all too dangerous.

When I complained, my mother reminded me of her sister's accident. "I cry to think about how she suffered, and all because she insisted on jumping her horse over the stone wall behind our house. First she had the concussion, then the loss of memory, and worst of all, she ran wild with the boys. There was nothing your grandparents could do. They finally had to put her in an institution. For years I visited her there, always guilty that I didn't stop her from trying to jump that horse. That's why I won't let you take any unnecessary risks on the ice."

But I had a talent for skating. Soon I was good enough to become a competitive skater. And I wanted to. One day the instructor suggested to my mother that I take advanced lessons. Well, you can probably imagine what happened. She yelled at the teacher, saying he had disobeyed her instructions, and immediately stopped me from taking lessons. I can't even begin to tell you how angry I was. Not that it did any good. As usual, my father sided with my mother and that was the end of that.

When I was sixteen, I decided to kill myself. I had no friends. I believed my parents wanted to see me dead. And I thought I deserved to die. It seems strange to hear myself say that now, because I love my life and would never think of giving it up. But as a teenager I felt trapped, as if I were a butterfly who was smothering to death because there was no way out of the cocoon.

Believe me, killing myself was not an easy thing to do. Preparing for it meant giving up everything that mattered, so that when the time actually came there was nothing much of life left to live. My body began to feel strange, as though it could come apart easily, and sometimes it did. My mind followed suit; reading no longer interested me, my words didn't seem to make much sense even to me. I felt scared and empty. Toward the very end, I didn't even see the trees or hear the birds. Then, one spring morning, after my mother refused to let me learn how to drive, and without any thought at all, I walked into the bathroom, locked the door, and swallowed a bottle of pills.

I woke up in a hospital bed furious that I was still living. My mother had done it to me again. I would never be able to get away from her. I remember going back to sleep in a desperate attempt not to face my reality. But sleep made room for an old nightmare in which I was so small that my mother could carry me around in her big black bag, the one she took to go shopping. The bag frightened me, so I kept trying to claw my way out. I always woke up just as a big hand pushed me back into the darkness.

As it turned out, that hospital bed was in a loony bin, a psychiatric hospital. I'll never forget the day room on that very first morning. Still in a haze from the drugs I had overdosed on, everything, everyone, looked surreal. A girl appeared out of nowhere and stood almost nose to nose with me, while she made her teeth chatter to mimic my fear. I screamed and ran to the other side of the room, where I found myself next to another girl who stood against the wall holding both arms rigidly over her head. In the middle of the room two girls were pulling each other's hair. And I couldn't take my eyes off the bunches of keys that the staff carried around. I cried to them, "Please let me out. I'll be good. I promise that I'll be good. I'll never try to kill myself again."

But that didn't help. No one listened.

I stayed in that hospital for a full year. My room was in a small brick building called "Adolescent Girls," as though that in itself was an illness. It stood at the edge of the beautifully groomed grounds that surrounded the main building of this private psychiatric hospital. Twelve of us lived in the smaller building. We had a day room, a dining hall, and plenty of windows to let in the light. However, the doors were always locked and there were time-out rooms called "isolation."

I can still see my parents coming to visit for the first time. Walking across the broad expanse of lawn, they looked frightened and lost, my father's suit too small for his bulging stomach and my mother carrying that awful oversized black bag. We all met in Dr. Walker's office. He sat in front of his big desk, while I sat huddled in a corner of an overstuffed couch as close to him as I could get. My parents chose straight-backed chairs as far from us as they could get in that small room.

My mother began to complain about me almost as soon as we all sat down. "I know what's wrong with you," she said, jabbing the air with her index finger, "and no doctor will convince me otherwise. You're a stubborn, spoiled child, and nothing more. I know why you tried to kill yourself. It was to get back at me—just because I wouldn't give you driving lessons. Don't you understand, I did it for your own good?"

Turning and twisting a limp handkerchief, tears streaming down her scowling face, she added, "How could you do that to me? You're as reckless and stubborn as my sister was, and you know what happened to her! You of all people know how guilty I still feel about letting her get on that horse. And then all those years she spent in the State Hospital when she wouldn't even talk to me. Now you've added to my burden.

"Mark my words, Nancy, right now you're in a private hospital that's more like a country club, but if you don't watch out, you'll end up in a state institution just like my sister."

The room grew very quiet after that. It was as though we were all holding our breaths. Meanwhile, I carefully selected a strand of my dark brown hair, taking the time to play with it, and then, with a sharp jerk, pulled it out.

My mother's voice was loud and shook in response. "How can you do that to yourself? You're making yourself ugly!"

"What the hell do you care?" I retorted, surprised at the harshness in my voice. "You're just a liar, even if you are my mother. I know the real reason you wouldn't let me have driving lessons. You're always too drunk to drive me to class that time of day. For once in your life, tell the truth."

There was silence again while I chose another strand of hair and repeated the ritual. This time my father yelled, "Stop it, stop it," and lurched out of his chair to grab my hands.

I panicked, thinking he wanted to kill me. "*Get away, get away!*" I screamed. When he didn't stop, I began kicking and scratching, trying desperately to protect myself. That's when the doctor pressed the buzzer to call for help. An aid rushed in and held my arms behind my back while a nurse gave me an injection.

At first I blamed Dr. Walker for that injection. I thought he was siding with my parents against me, so I decided never to speak to him again. But after a while it dawned on me that the injection got me out of that room, away from my parents. And for the first time in my life I actually thought I might be able to have a life without them. I can't explain the importance of that discovery except to say that for me it was a revelation.

Over the next few months I began to change from a lost little girl who faced a lifetime of emptiness to a person with a future. It might be strange to hear that trying to kill myself could have such a result, but sometimes life is like that. Maybe you don't understand, but if you had been in that hospital, and felt what I felt, you would.

In the glow of that transformation, a new special friend appeared.

Her name was Gertrude. I liked her immediately. But when I told Dr. Walker about her, he got a worried look on his face and said neither she nor Max was real. "Stop thinking about her," he said. "Instead, concentrate on making friends with real people." Gertrude disappeared the very next day.

Her disappearance was a terrible disappointment. I didn't quite realize it, but I had been waiting for another special friend since Max died. And when she disappeared, I was left with the same lonely hole I felt when I lost him, and also the same urge to fill it. However, I learned another important lesson: If I wanted to be normal, I could not have my special friends. And at that time, more than anything in the world, I wanted to be normal.

I took Dr. Walker's advice and concentrated on befriending the girls on my floor. That wasn't an easy thing to do, given how wild and weird they were. In fact, it seemed impossible. So I found myself trying to help them instead. I can't tell you how excited that made me, how joyful. Soon helping became a passion, a reason for living. Somehow I knew I would never get married and have my own little baby. An ordinary life wasn't in the cards for me. Instead, I vowed to devote my life to helping others just like me. Not only that—I also understood that I didn't have to wait until I grew up. I could start that same day.

Do you remember the girl who stood against a wall and kept both arms raised rigidly above her head? I decided that she was the first one I was going to help. Each day I stood next to her, and even though she didn't talk to me, I talked to her. Once, after I made a joke, I caught a slight smile on her face. That's when I understood she was listening even though she didn't say anything.

Maybe it was just my imagination, but I got the idea that she kept her arms raised high because she was holding up the ceiling. So I told her I could do it, too, and demonstrated this by raising my own arms and scrunching my face to show that I was concentrating hard on keeping the ceiling up. She said nothing. I did it some more. She still said nothing.

Then, one evening while the rest of the girls were busy watching television, I asked if she trusted me enough to take down her arms and let me do the work for a while. Much to my amazement, that's exactly what she did! I stood there for quite a while, beaming with delight, my arms held high, my mind focused on the effort. When I got tired, I asked for her help, and with a smile, she raised her arms again.

Eventually I was pronounced well enough to leave the hospital. The social worker arranged for me to live with my mother's cousin, Estelle, the same woman we had visited with when I was learning to skate. She had never married, had no children, and taught in the local high school. Frankly, I was always a little afraid of her and worried that I wouldn't be able to live up to her expectations.

It was a spare and humorless life we lived together, no sweets, no music, no television, not many visitors. My parents pretty much left me alone. I think they were frightened of me. They didn't even visit. Both of them were drinking more steadily now that I was gone, and they rarely left their house. So much the better. More than anything in the world I wanted to be normal. I made friends, bought new clothes, and learned how to drive. In short, I became a regular, if shy, kid. The idea that some-day I would learn to help other people faded from my mind, maybe be-cause it reminded me of the past and the fact that I really wasn't normal. Nevertheless, I went on to college and studied computer science. When I graduated, I got an apartment and even found a job.

My life over the next twenty years was anything but exciting. The work was boring. Sitting at the same desk day after day and staring at a screen trying to make sense of numbers that held very little meaning for me was a torture. And my social life was dull—I didn't yet have the nerve to look into the eyes of any person I found interesting.

It's hard for me to talk about those years, perhaps because they were so barren. I was frightened of my own imagination, frightened enough to stay away from anything that would stimulate it, including people. Occasionally I thought of killing myself, but even that thought would disappear into the deadness of the next day.

And then, quite unaccountably, when I was forty-one years old, my first inner guide appeared. It happened during the middle of the night while I was worrying about all the work I had to do the next day. When sleep didn't come, I got up and settled myself at the kitchen table with a cup of tea. It was very quiet in my little apartment; even the cat was asleep.

Suddenly I heard someone. She spoke very quietly, almost in a whisper. "Please don't be afraid of me. I am your inner guide. You can depend on me. I'm here to listen to your worries and to offer you another kind of seeing, the seeing that comes through your intuition."

Once I got over the shock of her presence, I decided to ask her about my work problems. "Can you tell me what should I do at work tomorrow? I'm afraid I'll get confused and mess up."

"Please ask me questions that I can answer with a yes or no," she said. "Once I give you that simple answer, I can also offer some explanation."

"Okay," I said. "Shall I go in to work tomorrow?"

"Yes. You can do everything that's being asked of you. We have clear evidence for that conclusion, because you've done it many times before. You're a very good worker."

I felt comforted by her answer and soon went back to bed and fell asleep. When I awoke the next morning, I simply got up and went to work. I felt no doubt, no worry. And then I did all the supervisor wanted of me and more. My inner guide was right!

As you might guess, however, I did feel guilty about having a guide. I supposed it meant I really was crazy, but somehow I wasn't upset enough about that to tell her to go away. Still, I decided to be careful. I went to see Barbara, a therapist my acupuncturist recommended. Much to my surprise, she believed the appearance of my inner guide was evidence that I was spiritually gifted, not crazy! It was hard for me to believe her; after all, I was actually diagnosed as mentally ill when I tried to kill myself. But slowly the idea that I was spiritually gifted sank in.

I'm grateful that every so often, when I need to, I can still go see Barbara and ask, "Am I crazy?"

The night after I had my first therapy session, my inner guide came to me in a dream, which meant I could catch a glimpse, fuzzy though it was, of her appearance. She was classically beautiful, dignified, elegant in her long white dress. I felt thankful that, of all the people in the world, she had chosen me.

She was very explicit about our relationship in that dream. "You must understand that I can only visit if you ask for me. It's your choice whether you want me to come or not. Also, you must call for me in the middle of the night when you're quiet and ready for some hard concentration. Last, please prepare for my visit—organize any background information you think I might need and compose a question that I can answer with a yes or no."

I waited for a few days, trying to get very clear about what I wanted from my guide. Then, rousing myself in the middle of the night, I carefully, respectfully asked if she would visit. When I heard her say yes, I gave her some background information about my job, including how long I had been doing the same thing and how boring it was. I also talked about my fear of quitting and the old worry of running out of money.

"What do you think?" I asked. "Should I quit?"

"Yes," she said simply, much to my surprise.

"Don't I have to look for something else first?"

"No."

"Should I go back to school and study something new?"

"Yes. It's important that you stay true to your old dream. Learn how to help other people. I know you can do that. You're a woman of many talents. And by the way, don't worry about the money."

Well, this was information I hadn't expected. It wasn't practical. Sure, I wanted to change jobs, but I really didn't know what else to do. That dream of helping people was an adolescent fantasy. Certainly, I thought of going back to school, but what would I study and where would I find the money?

"This doesn't make sense," I said to myself. "Get yourself back to reality, Nancy. You're going crazy."

Even though my therapist kept urging me to be patient, saying that I didn't know what would unfold, I put my inner guide back in the closet and tried to forget about the whole thing. But then my cousin Estelle died of a heart attack. The woman who had offered me a home after my stay in the hospital was no more. I cried for her, feeling even more alone in the world. Would anything good ever happen to me? Was I fated to live this muted dream of a life? The ache inside me grew ever stronger and I felt sure nothing could heal it. That's when I decided if there wasn't any change by my next birthday, I would kill myself. I had just three months to change my life.

A few weeks later our family lawyer called and said that Estelle had left me an inheritance. I had enough money to pay for school!

"Oh my God," I realized, "my inner guide was right. She told me not to worry about money and I didn't listen. How could I have been so foolish as to send her away?"

Would she ever visit me again? I wasn't sure. Still, I prepared myself meticulously for a visit, got up in the middle of the night, and waited for a few hours. About a week later, she came. The first thing I did was apologize for my disrespect. I was embarrassed by my disbelief. She was quick to forgive.

Then I told her about Estelle and the inheritance and asked for her advice. "Do you think I should go to school?"

"Yes," she replied. "You have a talent for helping people and you'll be a healer one day, if you aren't too afraid. There's a book about healing I would like you to read. It will help you face your fears."

Much to my surprise, the next morning I found that very book under a pile of books on the floor near my desk. And when I read the introduction, I learned that the author was the founder of a school for healers. Amazingly, I was being shown the way!

"Forget about being normal," I said to myself. "My inner guide is a gift and I will follow her to the ends of the universe."

However, a quiet voice inside added, "As long as you don't go crazy."

When I told my guide about that voice, she said not to worry. "By all means, do not silence it. Welcome whatever inner voices emerges, even those that are doubting and hateful. They need your close and critical attention. You have a lot to learn from all of them. It will take years, but eventually the voice that says you're crazy will grow so faint you'll barely make it out.

"There will also be other fully embodied guides just like me who will come to you. They can teach you much more about healing. Most important, if you learn to trust in our wisdom, you will learn to trust in yourself."

So I packed up my belongings, moved to Colorado, and became a student at the International School for Psychic Healers. I'm sure it's not surprising for you to hear that I was terribly scared and sure that I would fail miserably. I think I would have, if it wasn't for my guide. I couldn't have made it through without her. There were lectures, tests, and real life demonstrations. In each class we paired up with other students to practice healing techniques while our supervisors watched. These practice sessions were the most frightening of all, but I learned I could ready myself by asking my guide to help. Each time I would find that quiet space, put myself into a trance, and ask for a visit. Without fail, she came and told me exactly what to do. We were a team and would always be so.

Others began to notice how centered I was during a healing and how accurate my interventions. I became one of the most outstanding students. People thought I had a gift. Secretly, however, I knew that I really didn't understand what I was doing. No matter how much reassurance I got, I felt like an impostor, a fake. The fact that other students seemed to know even less than I did offered some solace, but not enough. I kept thinking it was my guide who was doing the work, not me. Often I thought of dropping out, but my guide kept assuring me that one day I would come to believe in my powers.

After graduation, I moved to Philadelphia and began my practice. Many people came to see me, perhaps because I had a reputation as a healer who got results. When I presented at conferences or went to workshops, well-known healers respected my work. Colleagues and teachers from my school asked for my help. My practice quickly grew. The truth remained, however, that my reputation was growing faster than my belief in myself, and I didn't know what to do about it. Even my guide couldn't help. Something had to happen to make me more sure of myself.

And it did. A woman called saying that her husband, Jim, was in the hospital and dying from cancer of the stomach. She was terribly upset and anxious that I help out quickly, so I decided to visit Jim that very day. First, however, I consulted my guide. She suggested that I listen very carefully to what Jim had to say even though he was in a coma.

Most important, I was to make sure he wasn't frightened of me.

I was very careful to do just that. First I stood very quietly at the foot of his bed, expecting he would know of my presence. Then I introduced myself and asked for permission to sit down. Of course he didn't answer, but I sensed that I should place my chair right near the door, as far from the bed as I could. From that distance I asked him to tell me what was happening. Without words he let me know about his illness and how afraid he was of dying. Soon he allowed me to move closer so I could use my hands to explore his body, although of course I didn't actually touch him. I was feeling for problems in the flow of his energy. Sure enough, I felt intense heat as my hands passed over his stomach. I knew immediately the cancer was producing it.

What to do next wasn't exactly clear to me. But I did know that any healing, regardless of the nature of the illness, had to be done with deep compassion. So I used all my senses to see and hear and feel into Jim. Only then could I really know him. Only then could I sense when he was ready to let go of whatever was keeping him ill. I sat quietly for a long time, listening, feeling, seeing.

Without words I suggested that he breathe gently and relax into his coma rather than trying to escape it. The coma was natural, I explained, and had a purpose. I promised to watch over him and give him all the help he needed. Also, I would keep working on his problem at home, throughout the night. Somewhere inside I heard him thank me.

As soon as I could after I got home, I asked my guide if my information about Jim was correct. "Yes and no," she said. "Explore his body again in your mind as you sit here, and go very slowly as you pass through his chest."

Sure enough, I found a second hot spot in his lungs.

I asked if I had any chance of healing him.

"Yes," she said. "With great compassion and little hope."

There was something very sad in her voice, so I went deep inside myself, slowed my breathing, and waited patiently, very quietly, until I heard from her.

Finally she asked: "What is it you want from me?"

"Can I succeed at saving him?"

"No, I'm afraid you can't. He will die."

"Should I do the healing anyway?"

"Yes. Never deny someone your good will."

And so I did the work while sitting quietly in my kitchen.

The next day Jim's wife called me. He had revived miraculously in the middle of the night, right around the time I had finished the healing. Sobbing, she said they were able to convey their love for each other and say good-bye. By morning he had stopped breathing. She was tremendously thankful for all I had done.

I cried for a long time after that telephone conversation. I did have the gift of seeing! And I could use that gift to help others! There was no need to doubt myself so much. I actually achieved the goal I had set for myself years ago in the hospital: to devote my life to helping people just like me. Only now I understand that I became pregnant at that moment—and finally, years later, gave birth to a healer.

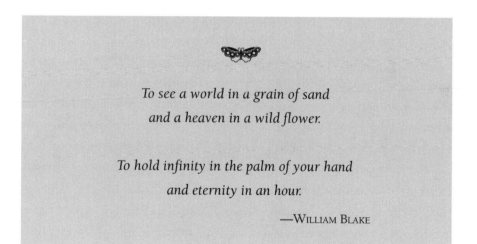

To see a world in a grain of sand
and a heaven in a wild flower.

To hold infinity in the palm of your hand
and eternity in an hour.

—William Blake

STRETCHING MIND TO ITS OUTER LIMITS

"There are more things in heaven and earth, Horatio, than are dreamt of in your philosophy," Shakespeare wrote about four hundred years ago. His admonishment is still relevant today; our commitment to everyday reality causes us to miss much of what goes on in the world around us. It's not as though we don't know there's a lot of "stuff" out there we cannot directly sense; we understand that waves of sound and light energy come in frequencies we cannot see or hear. We know DNA exists in every single cell of every living being on this earth, even though it's too small for most of us to see or touch. And we don't say scientists are irrational when they hypothesize that there's a black hole within our Milky Way that can't be seen but has a mass that is millions of times the mass of our sun. It's supposed to be the gravitational core of our galaxy, keeping objects, including our sun and its planets, from flying apart. Nor do we blink when scientists suggest that the subatomic particle called a neutrino has the capacity to move directly through material objects, much like a ghost through a door. There are things in the world that go against our common understanding. And still we hold on to the idea that *only* what we can see and touch exists.[1]

Our physical world is also constantly changing. Scientists tell us that the universe is expanding in some places and contracting in others. Suns burn out; galaxies are born and die. Given astronomical time, the sky is in constant flux. Given geological time, mountains rise and fall. Given human time, cultures appear and disappear.

Our social world is also impermanent. What we call *reality* actually is a perspective that shifts from person to person. Listen to two people describe the same car accident, or the same marital conflict, and it's soon apparent that interpretations of reality vary between people and over time. We see through the filter of our particular interpretive capacity.

Even the reliability of written history is uncertain. Deconstructionists (a group of contemporary philosophers) point out that the events historians write about, and the people they identify as key actors in those events, are chosen because of biases.[2] For example, males have played major roles in almost all historical accounts, and of course most historians have also been male. In recent years, however, more women have begun writing history, so history itself is changing; now the role of women in creating culture is being highlighted. Histories now include accounts of women's work, including planting, cooking, and child-rearing. But these accounts are also biased. Every single filter available to us, including Nancy's, is a bias, a perspective. And they're all true, in the sense that they bring to light another slice of this very complex world we live in.

Buddhists use the word *impermanence* to describe a reality that is in flux, that is constantly creating itself. Even the self is described as impermanent—as an ever changing flow of information from the very six senses by which we know the world, including ourselves. Within the Buddhist vocabulary, this perception is called *no-self*. It's a term that grows out of the Buddhist fondness for mystery. As you will see, *no-self* is less of a mystery than it seems.[3]

To explain, let's start with the conventional belief that the self is permanent: a stable, unchanging entity within each person. This idea, commonplace though it is, doesn't quite fit with commonplace experience—and yet it's very important to us. For example, if we detect a difference between how we act around the postman and how we act around the doctor, we might think something is wrong, that we should maintain an unchanging, unitary self. That's the conventional belief. Actually, serious problems arise if we hold on to the stable, the permanent, too tightly. Then we're shocked by creativity that threatens the conventional—a child who sees an imaginary friend, or perhaps paints a purple sun and an orange face, can become suspect, dangerous, or even crazy.

Often people assume the self is one with the body and then expect both to be stable. But from the perspective of impermanence, it doesn't make sense to look for a stable self in the body because the body itself is ever changing. Sometimes people assume that the stable self dwells in our consciousness. But from the perspective of impermanence, that doesn't work either, because the phenomenon we call consciousness is ever fleeting; we actually move in and out of awareness continually. As it turns out, wherever we look, the stable, unchanging self is not to be found. This was the Buddha's great discovery. When he talked of *no-self*, he meant to say that, even in our conventional world, impermanence reigns; the self is not an entity but, rather, an activity.

Verbs replace nouns when we see through the lens of impermanence; rather than using the noun *self*, we use the verb *selfing*. Even God becomes a verb as the emphasis shifts from creation to creating. Seeing through the lens of impermanence is a radical shift from our commonplace view of reality. For those who have a direct experience of this insight, the world can also flow.[4]

When we learn to live with impermanence, the activity of selfing allows for ongoing creativity. We see ourselves ever changing—being gentle and becoming angry, being absurd and becoming mundane. Selfing arises and fades in many forms. This doesn't mean we need to believe everything people say about their extraordinary experiences; it's simply a matter of staying open to the possibility that there's more in heaven and earth than we ever dreamt of.

Now let's think about a brown-haired, blue-eyed little girl named Nancy, maybe three or four years old, who couldn't find a place for herself in the "real" world of her family. Picture her in her favorite hiding places, secreted away in the kneehole of a desk or under a table, dreaming up a friend who was more *there* for her than the big people walking around. In itself, that's nothing remarkable. Many children create imaginary friends. But when Nancy began to talk to these figures in front of her parents, they became frightened and grasped desperately for a stable reality, one they could see and touch. And they communicated that fear to their daughter.

In her early years Nancy fought for the right to have her own reality, her own inner life, and it almost killed her. The hospital that she found herself in offered many things, including safety from her family; but perhaps most important, it offered her the experience of empathetically joining with the girl who was holding up the ceiling. Here was someone else who saw what others couldn't, and she also was labeled crazy. Quite remarkably, Nancy didn't laugh at her. Instead, she accepted the girl's perception of reality, and to Nancy's great surprise, that acceptance helped. It was a foretaste of the healer's art.

Unfortunately, the hospital also taught Nancy that she couldn't have her particular inner life and still be considered sane. And the institution, with its doctors in white coats and jangling bunches of keys, was a force too powerful to resist. So she chose the doctor's definition of reality and gave up her inner life. That led to many depressed and empty years.

But there was a fire glowing inside Nancy. Her strange dreams and voices persisted and often led to the panic that came when she believed she was going crazy. Finally, however, in midlife she was ready, and so she sensed the presence of her inner guide. That's when she came to see me.

From the first time we met, I was struck by the energy and the intensity Nancy brought to her search, and how much she suffered. Sitting across from her, I cried tears of remorse and anger. *Do no harm* is such an important mantra for a therapist, and yet, often without any intention, harm is done. Thankfully, there have been, and still are, great humanistic minds focused on the effort to heal the psyche. But the limitations of psychological theory have led many therapists to reject an exploration of the inner world in favor of simple behavioral change or drugs. And so, out-of-the-ordinary spiritual or mystical experiences are more suspect—if not feared. Seeing that which others do not see can be too quickly labeled a symptom of psychosis. Certainly, psychosis exists, and it needs to be treated appropriately. But there is also something called a spiritual path, and there are spiritual emergencies—those moments when the everyday world loosens its hold and people experience a different reality before they're ready for it. Labeling that experience *mental illness* does harm. I was grateful for the opportunity to help Nancy undo that harm.

It was clear that accepting the existence of Nancy's inner guide, who was a loving presence in her life, was essential for her well-being. So when Nancy came into therapy one day upset because she had one of her recurring nightmares about getting caught in her mother's oversized black bag, we asked her inner guide to join us in a meditation. As we settled into the stillness, Nancy invited her guide to be present. Her guide agreed, and with great respect Nancy asked her what she could do to stop having the dream. We sat in the quiet waiting for a response. And then it came to Nancy: "Energy takes many forms, and sometimes a form is frightening. But there's no need for fear; it's just energy. And there's no need to stop the dream. Just watch." We both chuckled with pleasure.

Nancy received many gifts along the way, perhaps the most important among them being the capacity to accept her difference, the honing of her intuition, and an increasing power to see that which cannot be seen. Slowly she became a respected healer.

Our world is a great mystery. The way things come and go is much like the childhood game of peek-a-boo. Not only streams and mountains, but cultures, political systems, and healing practices are ever changing. Human beings are born and die. The wonder is that this impermanence makes room for everything else. And it also makes one particular life precious. Our hearts go out to the flower because its beauty comes and goes so quickly. Our minds blaze at the sight of a butterfly's wing shimmering in the sunlight because it is so fleeting. Impermanence is more than an abstract idea; it's a poignant miracle.

Imagine a rich cup of broth that is the width and breadth of the cosmos. Inside it, all phenomena happen. They arise, take shape, live out their own particular existence, and then melt back into the broth. People, birds, mountains, languages, religions, methods of healing arise, manifest in great and beautiful detail, and then melt away. In this cup of broth every living being, each language, every religion is precious and of equal value. It contains everything that is, including each and every one of us. Our ever-so-brief existence takes place within it. This broth is the home of the mystic. It is the place where the path toward wholeness leads us.

As you'll recall, the objects of awareness in Mindfulness Meditation are the six senses themselves: *hearing, seeing, tasting, smelling, feelings in the body,* and *thoughts in the mind.* Observing them with mindfulness and equanimity, we gain insight into experience.

In the first and second meditations, we meditated on feelings in the body. In the third and fourth meditations, we learned several ways of exploring internal conversation. Now we turn to another sense gate, namely, internal imaging.

To understand what I mean by internal imaging, look down at yourself for a moment; see your chest, your abdomen, your legs, your arms. Then close your eyes and try to catch a faint outline, a glimmer of what you just saw. That's internal imaging. If you watch for them, there are many images that pass before your eyes. Indeed, there's likely to be one for every thought you have.[5]

Studying any of the six senses in meditation, you can have direct experiences of impermanence. When you *hear* mindfully, you catch impermanence, whether it be in the sound of the tide or the wind as it ebbs and flows. When you *feel* mindfully, you sense how a pain in your body comes and goes. The attempt to *think* mindfully demonstrates how thoughts arise, gain clarity, and then fade away in an effortless flow. Even *seeing* mindfully illustrates impermanence—images and colors may very well arise and flow into each other on the screen in front of your closed eyes as you meditate.

As a child, Nancy could see and hear what others could not, and because no one was there to say that this was a natural occurrence, she got caught in fear. As she became wiser, she understood that the creative or out-of-the-ordinary also exists. Once she became aware of the flow of impermanence, she was even more likely to experience the creative or out-of-the-ordinary, whether it was a hint of an idea, the shadow of an image, or the echo of a sound. These were the very experiences she had dismissed as unreal or, worse still, crazy.

Impermanence is pure creativity. And everything, the tangible and intangible, material and spiritual, is included. It's a birthing, composing, transforming endeavor that shapes life itself.

The meditation that follows is one I learned from Shinzen years ago. It's an interesting introduction to impermanence. After a few moments of concentration practice, I'll ask you to close your eyes and place your awareness on the screen in front of your eyelids. Following Shinzen's instructions, if you see a well-defined image, label that *clear*.

Alternatively, the image might be so fuzzy or cloudy that you will wonder whether you imagined it. Much that goes on in our psyche is unclear, just the hint or even an idea of an image. Label that *subtle*.

There are times when you will see nothing at all or, instead, the amoebalike movement of colors on the screen in front of your eyes. Either is fine. Just enjoy the experience. And for our purposes, label that *nothing*.

As you will see, when you slow down the experience of seeing in meditation, you gain access to a range of experience we usually deny ourselves. However, if an image bubbles up from your psyche that bothers you, please give yourself permission to stop the meditation. You might even want to seek the advice of a counselor or a meditation teacher before you try it again. But most often, these images broaden and enrich your sense of what is and bring great beauty into your life.

So let's begin. Follow the meditation in the book or listen to it on the

CD. Make sure to have a timer by your side, and don't forget to take some notes on your experience of internal imaging. Use the memory prompt at the end of this chapter if you like.

"The only courage that is demanded of us [is to be open to] the most extraordinary, the most singular, and the most inexplicable that we may encounter . . ."

—RILKE

A Meditation on Seeing through the Lens of Impermanence

Settle into the body, and take several deep breaths.

Now calm your mind with the meditation called "A Meditation on Finding the Stillness." Set your timer for five minutes.

When you finish that meditation, open your eyes and look at the scene in front of you. Be aware of the floor . . . the walls . . . see the furniture.

Then close your eyes . . . and try to catch a glimpse of what you saw with your eyes open. This is internal image. If necessary, repeat this sequence during the meditation. It will help you learn how to see internal image.

*Now, with your eyes shut and your head facing forward, shift the focus of awareness to what lies to the **left** of you. See or imagine the floor . . . the walls . . . chairs.*

*Let go of that, and make the focus of awareness what lies to the **right** of you. See or imagine the floor, walls, ceiling . . . chairs . . . lamps . . .*

*Then shift your awareness to the scene that lies **behind** you. See or imagine the furniture, the walls, the ceiling.*

*This time, see or imagine what lies **below** you . . . the floor . . . a rug. Be aware of how image after image arises . . . manifests . . . and fades, as it is replaced by another.*

Last, be aware of what lies **above** *you. See or imagine the ceiling . . . the lights.*

Our direct experience of the world is as an ever changing series of sensations. Breathe deeply and allow for the flow.

❀

Let's go through this experience once more. This time give yourself the freedom to stretch your imagination so it goes through walls. With your eyes closed, be aware of what lies in **front** *of you . . . the floor . . . the walls . . . the furniture. Now imagine what lies outside of the room in front of you . . . another room . . . a sidewalk . . . a garden. What do you see?*

Shifting, place your awareness on what lies to the **right** *of you . . . floor . . . walls . . . ceiling . . . Then stretch with your imagination to imagine what lies outside the room . . . another room? With walls? A ceiling? A floor? Perhaps, you can catch the flow of cars moving down the closest avenue or highway.*

Shifting again, be aware of what lies to the **left** *of you . . . floor . . . walls . . . ceiling. Then stretch beyond the room . . . perhaps to the edge of your town or city . . . to where there are fields or mountains or waters. Where does your imaginataion take you?*

This time, shift your awareness to what lies **behind** *you. Stay there for a while . . . and stretch beyond the room.*

Now shift to the scene that lies below you. Use your imagination to move into the ground **below** *. . . perhaps to the other side of this round globe.*

Last, with your eyes closed, be aware of what lies **above** *you. Use your imagination to see the sky . . . with its billions of stars. Be aware of how one image fades as another emerges.*

Take five minutes to repeat this part of the meditation.

❀

When you're ready, return to the memory of the trouble you named in the first meditation. Keep your awareness on the screen in front of your eyes, and imagine or see a fuzzy image of someone who is part of your trouble, or perhaps . . . a scene associated with your trouble.

If no image arises . . . enjoy the quiet.

If, along with an image, body sensations emerge—feelings that are associated with emotions such as anger or shame—be aware . . . and gently return to the image . . . or the flow of images . . . or the peace that comes with no image.

Perhaps you sense the fleeting nature of your trouble as you know it through this sense gate.

Set your timer for ten minutes and continue this part of the meditation

❁

And now it's time to end this meditation. With your eyes still closed, sit for a few more moments. And congratulate yourself for directly experiencing the flow of impermanence that's built into life.

Slowly open your eyes. As you move through the day, be aware of how scene after scene arises, manifests, and fades away. This is an important insight into how this world of ours is put together.

May all beings know impermanence.

Training for Awareness

1. Repeat the meditation called "A Meditation on Finding the Stillness."

2. Contact internal image. See the scene in front of you, to the right, behind, to the left, below, and above.

3. See the scenes in all directions as you imagine they look outside the room, beyond what you can ordinarily see.

4. Recall the trouble you're working on. Keep contact with internal image.

Six

Strawberries

There's an old Zen tale about a monk who went for a walk one day only to realize that he was being stalked by a tiger. He ran away as quickly as he could, but the tiger was in hot pursuit and rapidly gained ground. Coming to a precipice, the monk grabbed hold of a wild vine and swung himself down over the edge. Hanging there, he saw the tiger greedily sniffing at him from above, and another tiger waiting to eat him should he fall. Then he realized the vine that held him was being gnawed at by two small mice with big teeth. At that moment his eyes fell on a beautiful red strawberry growing just within his reach.

What was he to do? Instantly the answer came; holding the vine in one hand, he plucked the strawberry with the other. How sweet it tasted!

As the monk was about to die, he knew the fleeting nature of all life. The exquisite but all too brief taste of the strawberry was an expression of his insight into impermanence. He suggests appreciating the immediacy of the moment, because that is essentially what we have.

With this in mind, let's pause in the flow of stories so we can reflect on this effort to explore the healing of emotions. Where have the women's stories taken us? Were there strawberries along their paths? Where do the meditations lead the rest of us? Can we catch a glimpse of a path toward wholeness?

Two healing traditions come together in Mindfulness Psychotherapy. Each offers its own answers to the questions posed here, yet they're also quite similar. The first, psychotherapy, is our homegrown, Western rendition of healing. It helps us uncover the veils of identity we acquire along the way—be they in our life story, the habit-driven patterns that propel us, or the emotions that drive us. A course of psychotherapy loosens those veils of identity and so makes room for exploring other ways of being. The second discipline, Mindfulness Meditation, teaches how to use awareness to scrub clean the senses—seeing, hearing, tasting, smelling, feelings in the body, and thoughts in the mind. As a result, we know experience more directly, beyond the veils of identity. This makes our lives richer and at the same time simpler and clearer.

Tozan, a famous Zen master, offers an image that for me describes the relationship between the two disciplines: "The blue mountain is the (parent) of the white cloud. The white cloud is the (offspring) of the blue mountain. All day long they depend on each other, without being dependent on each other. The white cloud is always the white cloud. The blue mountain is always the blue mountain." Psychotherapy and Mindfulness Meditation are much like the white cloud and the blue mountain as they come together in Mindfulness Psychotherapy. They depend on each other, but each has its own trajectory.[1] Together they prepare us to choose the strawberry when life is most difficult. The taste is enlightening.

And now on to our questions.

WHERE HAVE THE WOMEN'S STORIES TAKEN US?

Marcel Proust once wrote, "The real voyage of discovery consists not in seeing new landscapes but in having new eyes." We learn just that from the women; their voyages of discovery consisted not in finding new selves but in soaking their everyday selves with awareness. As it turns out, this simple but very difficult practice heals emotions. And trouble is often the starting point.

Each of the five women we have visited so far used the following guidelines to find their way—not as definitive directions, but as hints or clues that shed some light. These same guidelines are built into the meditations described in this book.

NAMING TROUBLE

Even though being aware of trouble is essential to healing, many people avoid this knowing; indeed, they are spooked by trouble. It's as though the emperor has no clothes on as he parades before us, and no one sees his naked body—because we're afraid to face the fact of his nakedness. Naming is an act of awareness. It opens the door to many different kinds of healing activity. But it's very hard for some people. Maria, for instance, spent years not knowing that she was sexually abused by her father. Once she knew it, her life began to change.

NAMING THE EMOTIONS THAT COME WITH TROUBLE

Trouble is built into the nature of life. In that sense, it intrudes upon us from the outside. The loss of a loved one or the discovery of an illness impinges on us and our sense of well-being. On the other hand, emotions are internal; they bubble up from the feeling core of our being. To know our emotions, awareness must be directed inside, toward them. Often this is hard to do, because we live with the pervasive belief that focusing on our emotions increases their strength. In truth, awareness exposes the reality that all emotions, regardless of the kind, arise, reach their peak, and then fade away. It's only if we clutch, and so resist, them that they hang on. I relied upon this natural restorative pattern to help heal the emotions of the women in this book. It was their resistance to emotions that needed to change.

CULTIVATING COMPLETE ACCEPTANCE

Many people who can name their trouble still continue to maintain it, perhaps for as long as a lifetime. It's as though they have an on/off awareness switch installed in their psyches. At moments when the switch is turned on, they're aware of their trouble. When the switch is off, it's as though the trouble doesn't exist. Unfortunately, the switch is usually in the off position, and they live their lives unaware that their marriage is failing or that the next drink will lead to many others.

This is only half of the problem; these people often use that on/off switch to deal with their emotions as well. It's one thing to name an emotion; it's quite another to completely accept its existence and so experience it fully. For instance, a person may be able to name her fear but unable to listen to the panicky thoughts and feel the jittery, quivering sensations in her body. If she could do so, healing would become more likely. Cultivating a complete acceptance of trouble and its emotions is a radical endeavor. It leads to a clarity of mind and a fullness of heart.

DEVELOPING EQUANIMITY

Every one of the skills taught in Mindfulness Psychotherapy circles around the capacity for equanimity, the balanced state of mind that is not thrown off course by the next emotion. Naming trouble, naming the emotions triggered by trouble, and completely accepting trouble and its emotions all rely on the capacity to be matter-of-fact and unprejudiced. The fact is, awareness by itself is not enough to heal emotions. For healing to take place, we need a foundation from which to deal with life—and that's what equanimity offers.

Equanimity is formally taught in many spiritual traditions. It can also be cultivated through sustained athletic activity, immersion in music, or gardening. It's a radical endeavor that leads to a clarity of mind and a fullness of heart.

EXPLORING THE MIND/BODY PROCESS

Each of the women explored her mind/body process. The women used their awareness to explore feelings in the body, thoughts in the mind, and the images that arose in night dreams, daydreams, and everyday life.

Tanya used this process to penetrate the grief that came with Chuck's death. Eventually, she felt that grief in her body, heard it in her mind, and saw manifestations of it at night. She learned to watch the waves of her grief rise and fall with equanimity. And the sound of the blues was the strawberry she plucked along the way.

Kate's challenge was to reject death and, instead, deal with her trouble—marital abuse. The *NO* she heard herself say when she tried to get out of bed to greet her husband was her insight, her strawberry. It awakened her to the emotion of anger. Exploring her mind/body process, she gathered enough strength not only to leave her husband but also to survive a serious depression.

Laura's trouble was mirrored by our culture's trouble: homophobia. Her challenge was to live authentically. To do that, she explored the mind/body process that combined her sexual interest with shame. The strawberry she plucked took the form of a new sexual awakening and newfound self-acceptance.

Maria had to face the trouble of sexual abuse in her childhood. It came with a particularly harsh judging mind. Once she learned how to sustain an awareness of her angry internal talk and accept the reality of her self-hatred, these emotions had less power. Not that her self-hatred was dispelled forever. Such a strong emotion comes in waves, hopefully weaker over time, throughout the stages of a life. As for her strawberry, it was the birth of a little baby called Maria.

And last, Nancy used Mindfulness Meditation to accept a personal reality—the existence of beings that cannot be seen in everyday life—that our culture considers evidence of insanity. She explored the mind/body process that included the fear of going crazy, and dispelling that fear, she went on to become a healer. Along the way, she gave herself permission to pick a strawberry that took the form of an inner guide.

FORMING AN OBSERVING SELF

Every one of these women developed this capacity to observe herself in everyday life. Her ongoing observation became an effort to increase her awareness of the nature of life as it is. That corner of the mind became a way of life.

PRACTICING COMPASSION

Ultimately, healing comes through the kind of love we call compassion, and it begins when that love is turned inward, toward the self. Over the years, I have learned that the emergence of self-love is a sign that healing is taking place. When a woman was able to hear me congratulate her for having made progress, that was a good sign. Better still was when she could affirm one small but courageous step that she took toward healing. Compassion led the women to give back to others the insights, the love, and the caring they had given themselves.

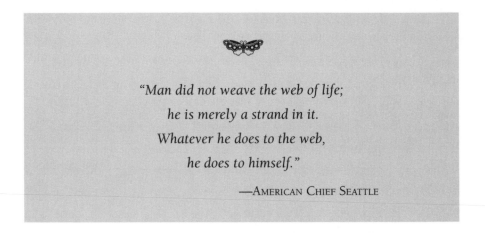

"Man did not weave the web of life;
he is merely a strand in it.
Whatever he does to the web,
he does to himself."

—AMERICAN CHIEF SEATTLE

WHERE DO THE MEDITATIONS LEAD US?

The meditations at the end of each chapter are tools we can use to heal troublesome emotions. As you know, Mindfulness Meditation teaches how to increase one's awareness of the senses. For our purposes, we focus on the three major sense gates: feelings in the body, thoughts in the mind, and internal imagery. This effort moves us away from content and toward a focus on the potency or the energy of a sensation.

In the first chapter we meditated on the sense gate that is the *body* and learned how to be still enough to actually be aware of it.

In the second chapter we learned how to scan the body for sensations that are part of an *emotion*—the tightness in the chest that signals anger, the lump in the throat that's a precursor to tears, or the flutter in the abdomen that might be fear.

In the third and fourth chapters we learned how to listen to the thoughts in the mind that we call *internal talk*. Doing these meditations, we first focused on developing the capacity for listening to internal talk, without paying attention to content. And then the instructions shifted so that the object of meditation became the content itself. That allowed us to develop the capacity to determine whether our internal talk was about planning for the future, judging ourselves or others, memory, or fantasy. We also focused on becoming aware of the judging mind, that terrible propagator of pain.

This led to chapter 5 and the focus on *internal imagery,* along with the possibility of an insight into impermanence. We learned to watch the screen in front of our eyes for those fuzzy, cloudy impressions that we can barely see. For many of us, these are the most fleeting of the sense impressions. Watching for them, one can't avoid sensing the evanescent nature of that which is—what we call *impermanence.*

As you shall soon see, we're now ready to use all three sense gates in one meditation. This is another step toward learning the tools with which to explore the mind/body process. Over time, the tools will provide us with the insights that lead to growth and healing.

Can We Catch a Glimpse of a Path toward Wholeness?

Let's review what Mindfulness Psychotherapy has suggested about the nature of the path toward wholeness, recognizing, however, that the only way to know this path is through direct experience.

- *Trouble is often the gateway to the path toward wholeness.* If we dig down through the layers of insecurity, hurt, loneliness, pain, and fear that exist inside most of us, we're likely to find still other layers of the same. If we don't run away, we might be motivated to use practices such as psychotherapy and meditation to dig still deeper. Living close to pain and suffering, sensing the whole of it, the reality of it, day after day, year after year, we take a step toward wholeness and the love that comes with it.

- *The path teaches compassion* for all beings, both those caught in illusion and those on the path. Compassion is a healing potion; feeling it, we take extra special care of ourselves and every other being on this earth of ours.

- *The path requires equanimity.* This is the capacity to be close to our troublesome emotions and, at the same time, distant enough to loosen their hold. Equanimity offers insight into two fundamental characteristics of the larger whole: that everything and everyone has a place, and we're all of equal value.

- *Impermanence or change is built into the path.* Indeed, the learning is that permanence is impossible. The reality is that everything comes and goes. This gives seekers the opportunity to be transformed as they follow the path toward wholeness.

- *The self is not separate.* Perhaps the hardest challenge of all is to undo our belief in a separate self that is clearly detached from other beings and the natural world. Mindfulness Psychotherapy leads us beyond our individual identities into a deep connection with the whole.

Let's take a moment to explore this connection, beginning with a story told by Thich Nhat Hanh. He says:

I learned that to make peanut butter cookies, you mix all the ingredients to prepare the batter, and then you put each cookie onto a cookie sheet using a spoon. I imagined that the moment each cookie leaves the bowl of dough and is placed onto the tray, it begins to think of itself as separate. You, the creator of the cookies, know better, and you have a lot of compassion for them. You know that they are originally all one, and that even now, the happiness of each cookie is still the happiness of all the other cookies. But they have developed a range of discriminative perceptions, and suddenly they set up barriers between themselves. When you put them in the oven they begin to talk to each other: 'Get out of my way. I want to be in the middle. I am brown and beautiful and you are ugly! Can't you please spread a little in that direction?'[2]

Not only do we want to be separate, but we also paradoxically want to belong. In fact, the experience of being separate precipitates a *craving to belong.* That craving leads us to make myriad distinctions about the groups we want to belong to. And with each distinction comes a judgment—good or bad, right or wrong, subtle or blatant.

This brings us to the *we-against-them* illusion. Caught in this illusion, it seems that we can have more of this belonging if we deny it to others—those whom we deem to be outcasts, savages, or aliens. The list can also include animals, trees, even the earth itself. These others, whom we already consider to be lesser than we, are as a result denied the compassion we expect for ourselves. Of course, ours is not the only culture that is caught in the *we-against-them* illusion. Given the mass destruction that's taken place within the past century, we humans certainly take it to an extreme. And so it is that the illusion of a separate self leads to tremendous suffering in the world.

Fortunately, there are many people across the globe who see through these illusions. These people are motivated to seek the path toward wholeness. Indeed, they *are us.* Learning to know holistically, we understand that the living system called the earth is made up of everyone and everything, and we can survive only if the rest of the earth survives. We are a power of untold dimensions.[3]

In the following meditation we'll experiment with accessing all three sense gates. This gives a more complete experience of an emotion; as such, it's more likely to call forth moments when we know holistically. It's preparation for seeing the strawberries along the path.

During the first part of the meditation, focus your awareness on the *body*, be it the touch of your clothes or the feeling of tension in the chest. The challenge is to keep as continuous an awareness or contact with the body as you can.

Then turn your attention to the place where you see *internal imagery.* Most people see it on the screen that's created when you close your eyes. Remember, one way to identify internal imagery is to open your eyes and look at your body as it is. Then close your eyes and see some rendition of that same image of yourself. It may be fuzzy and cloudy, or it may be clear. Again, the challenge is to keep as continuous a contact as you can with the place where you see internal imagery.

In the third part of the meditation, make the place where you hear *internal talk* the object of meditation. Recall that one way to identify internal talk is to place your awareness in the area of your head where you tend to hear talk. Then say your name silently to yourself, and determine where you're hearing the sound: in your two ear canals, someplace toward the back of your head, or somewhere else.

Put these together and we have what Shinzen calls *BIT*—body . . . image . . . talk—as the object of the meditation. We will, in fact, experiment with putting two of the sense gates together, namely, body sensations and internal images, internal images and internal talk, and finally, internal talk and body sensations. Or, we might say, body-image, image-talk, talk-body.

As you will see in the next chapter, the BIT meditation that follows is helpful in deconstructing the mind/body process that's associated with troublesome emotions.[4] In this chapter we will concentrate on learning the meditation technique.

Now settle in and get ready for the meditation. Read all the instructions through once, and then read and do each section. Use the brief outline in the box to jog your memory.

"We do not receive wisdom, we must discover it for ourselves, after a journey through the wilderness, which no one else can make for us, which no one can spare us, for our wisdom is the point of view from which we come at last to regard the world."

—MARCEL PROUST

A Meditation on the Nature of Self

Take a few deep breaths and let the body settle. Allow a small smile to spread across your face. Sense the stillness. The object of this first part of the meditation is simply to keep continuous contact with the body.

Begin by letting your awareness float freely in the body. Perhaps you will sense the touch of your shirt on your back . . . the heat of your hands as they hold each other. Maybe you will feel the tightness that comes with anger . . . or a flutter that comes with fear. Label the location of each awareness . . . knee . . . hands . . . face . . . stomach.

If thoughts arise, make them background and simply return to the body.

If sounds intrude, make them background and simply return to the body.

Set your timer for five minutes and keep continuous contact with the body.

❧

*The object of this second part of the meditation is to keep continuous contact with that place where you see **internal imagery**. You can learn what internal imagery is by opening your eyes for a moment and looking at your own body. Then close your eyes and see if you can catch a glimpse of the body, be it clear or a fuzzy cloudlike resemblance.*

Keep contact with the place where you see internal imagery. Perhaps you will see nothing . . . that's all right . . . just enjoy the rest. Maybe you will see the play of color or light on the screen in front of your eyes. Simply watch. Remember, the object of this part of the meditation is simply to keep contact with that place where you see internal images.

Perhaps as you watch you will see a clear, almost photographic image. If so, label it clear.

Maybe you will sense some kind of cloudy image, a vague outline that is so fleeting you may doubt it occurred. If so, label it subtle.

If you see no image, or if you see the interplay of colors . . . for our purposes, label that nothing . . . and enjoy the peace.

Set your timer for five minutes and keep contact with that place where you see internal imagery.

❧

The object of this third part of the meditation is to keep continuous contact with that place where you hear **internal talk**.

When you're ready, place your awareness in your ear canals, or wherever you tend to hear your internal dialogue. Then listen.

Often, just placing your awareness on internal talk makes it stop. That's fine. Just label that none *. . . and enjoy the peace.*

Or, you may hear the judging mind . . . or the planning mind . . . loud and clear. For our purposes in this meditation . . . the content doesn't matter. Just say clear.

Again, you may hear bits and pieces of words that often make little sense. Just say subtle. *Keep the focus of your awareness in your ear canals or wherever you hear internal talk.*

If body sensations interfere, simply return to the place where you hear internal talk. And have patience.

If you get bored or impatient . . . try to let those feelings be background . . . and return to the place where you hear your internal dialogue.

Set your timer for five minutes and continue this part of the meditation.

❁

The object of the next three parts of the meditation is to hold two of the sense gates in awareness at the same time.

Place your awareness in the **body** *. . . and then shift some part of your awareness to the place where you might see an* **internal image**. *Remember, the object of this meditation is to keep contact with the two sense gates as continuous as you can. Feel . . . watch.*

Take five minutes to keep contact with the body and the place where you might see an internal image.

❁

When you return . . . keep contact with the place where you might see an **internal image**. *And then place some of your awareness in that place where you hear* **internal talk**.

Try to hold in awareness . . . both the place where you might see an internal image and the place where you might hear internal talk. Watch . . . listen.

Take five minutes and continue this part of the meditation.

❀

*Now, keep some of your awareness in the place where you hear **internal talk** and some of your awareness on **body** sensations.*

See if you can hold both sense gates in awareness at the same time. Listen . . . feel.

Take five minutes and keep your awareness on the place where you hear internal talk . . . and be aware of any body sensations that arise.

❀

This time, set your timer for five minutes and go from one combination to another . . .

> *body sensations and internal images*
> *internal images and internal talk*
> *internal talk and body sensations*

Feel and watch . . . watch and listen . . . listen and feel. Feel and watch . . . watch and listen . . . listen and feel. Feel and watch . . . watch and listen . . . listen and feel.

❀

Last, set your timer for five minutes and hold all three senses in awareness: body sensations . . . internal images . . . internal talk.

Feel . . . watch . . . listen. Even if you can do this for only a brief moment, it's an important experience.

❀

When you're ready, open your eyes and sit quietly for a few moments. Congratulate yourself for staying with this meditative workout.

Perhaps you were able to meditate on the body more easily than on internal talk. Maybe you couldn't keep much contact with the place where you see internal images. It might be that the meditation as a whole feels tiring— too tiring. Many beginning meditators have the same experience. Please remember that simply making the effort is important. It takes courage and determination to continue . . . and practice will eventually allow you to find the strawberries that grow along the path.

May all beings know wholeness.

Training for Awareness

1. Be aware of the body. Let your awareness float freely on body sensations. Label locations.

2. Be aware of the place where you see internal images. Label *clear, subtle,* or *none.*

3. Be aware of the place where you hear internal talk. Label *clear, subtle,* or *none.*

4. Be aware of feelings in the body and the place where you see internal images.

5. Be aware of the place where you see internal images and the place where you hear internal talk.

6. Be aware of the place where you hear internal talk and be aware of feelings in the body.

7. Move from combination to combination: Body–Image, Image–Talk, Talk–Body.

Seven

Mae Is Changing the World

Mae, look at yourself—standing on the kitchen table with a butterfly net in your hand trying to catch a yellow canary while three children are babbling below and chocolate chip cookies are about to burn in the oven. Laughing out loud, I caught the canary, scrambled down from the table, got to the stove before the cookies burned, and showed Tommy and David, ages nine and four, how to spoon out the next batch of batter onto baking sheets.

Turning to take care of the baby, I heard a loud crash quickly followed by screams of terror. David had spilled the bowl of cookie dough on the floor and, carried away by that mishap, dumped an extra large spoonful of dough on Tommy's dark curly hair. In turn, Tommy made a snowball of dough and was about to throw the entire weight of his body behind a thrust aimed at David's nose. I reached them just in time.

"You're a cocksucker," little David shouted. "I hate you . . . "

"Cut out that language!" I yelled, outraged. "I've had it with the two of you. Apologize to each other. Right now!"

David's anger quickly collapsed into a puddle of tears and a quiet whimper. "Sorry, Tommy, I won't do it anymore."

I didn't ask what the "it" was, because I wasn't clear whether David

133

really knew, and this wasn't a time to find out; he was too upset. Meanwhile Tommy just stood there, bottom lip jutting out in a show of belligerent bravado, so I planted myself about a foot in front of him, crossed my arms, and glared back until he dropped the pose and apologized. Then I gave each a hug, two cookies, and a glass of milk.

Good work, even if I say so myself. Mornings like this, when I'm able to manage the kids' anger and pain, I'm proud to be a foster care mother. What better work than to take in broken children and make them whole! I'm their guardian angel, their protector, and I have enough magic dust in my pocket to make them grow up strong and healthy. But enough of that. Look at Tamika, almost two and a half but still rocking herself for comfort. She's too quiet— probably scared.

"Come on little one, let me clean you up and we'll go outside. I know you need comforting, and I can give it to you now." Settling into the swing under the old maple tree, I held her close and hummed the same lullaby I used to sing to my own daughter. *Poor sweet baby. She wasn't wanted and neither was I. She had an alcoholic father and so did I. It doesn't take too much effort for me to remember my father screaming and my mother cowering. Ugh! It still sends shivers through my spine. Probably Tamika has her own fuzzy bad memories. But now you have me, my little one, and I will make it better.*

The telephone rang; with babe in arms, I ran inside in time to hear Miss Peters, the case manager assigned to Tommy, announce that she was coming to see me this afternoon. "You still haven't sent me any of the July reports, Mae, and it's already August 20th. You're late again! Why can't you just fill them out? For heaven's sake, what's wrong with you?"

I felt my face grow warm with embarrassment. Truth to tell, I didn't even know where the forms were. Not that I hadn't looked. Last night, after the children were asleep, I actually spent a couple of hours rummaging through the piles of paper on my desk, in the kitchen, and on the dining room table, but to no avail. I never could get myself organized; it was a lifelong problem. So now I had to eat crow: "I'm sorry, Miss Peters, but I've misplaced the ones you sent me. I'd appreciate your bringing along another set."

"I should have known," she responded curtly. "It's just another example of how you can't keep anything straight. Yes, I'll bring them, and you'll fill them out this afternoon right in front of me. Otherwise, I'll never get them!" The phone clicked off.

A lump settled in my throat as if I wanted to cry and scream at the same time.

She's just like the rest of the case managers I've known—officious, bound to bureaucratic rules that often do more harm than good. No experience with kids, but she believes she knows what's best for them. She never talks to me about my work, but she thinks I don't know what I'm doing. Here I am, giving these children medicine that heals, and all she does is complain about paperwork!

In frustration, I opened the freezer door and served myself a big bowl of ice cream. But even that couldn't stave off the inevitable: I had to clean the house before this afternoon's visit. The agency had cleanliness rules, and I'd already been written up several times for failure to comply. Given the opportunity, Miss Peters would do it again. "Rules are rules," she often cackled.

At first it all seemed hopeless; just cleaning the kitchen could take the entire afternoon with kids around to get in the way. But when I told Tommy and David that Miss Peters was coming, they actually began picking up their toys in the living room while I worked in the kitchen. *What good kids! Why is it nobody appreciates them but me?*

It wasn't too long, however, before I heard Tamika complaining, so I called out to the boys, "From the sound of Tamika's voice I can only believe that one of you is bothering her."

David called back: "The pirates told me to do it."

"They told you to do what?"

"Take her toy," he answered.

"Tell those pirates not to give you such bad advice," I retorted playfully.

"I already did," said David, "but they wouldn't listen!"

I chuckled to myself. *Here's a comment that needs no response. David is developing a conscience of his own!*

The kids and I were well into the cleaning job when Miss Peters barged in, her high heels clicking down the center hall and into the kitchen. She was ever so thin in her blue business suit, her hair wrapped tightly, severely. Her cold gray eyes frightened me; they darted around the room, registering disapproval. *Damn her!*

Settling herself at the kitchen table, she immediately got down to the business of producing my delinquent reports. The boys offered her a cool glass of lemonade, which she abruptly refused. So they settled near us, on the floor, much like two sad little puppies. *Can't she see the children want a smile? What's the matter with her?*

As soon as the paperwork was finished, Miss Peters asked to speak to me outside, in the garden, where we could have some privacy. Moving toward the kitchen door, she pointed toward the boys and said sternly, "You better behave yourselves, or you're sure to hear from me!"

"I got a call from Tommy's mother yesterday," she launched in before we even sat down at the picnic table. "The woman was very upset. Tommy told her you were mean to him, that you often grab him and pull him around by the arm and you embarrass him in front of David. Tommy said one time you shook him so hard he began to cry." She added, "I asked David about it and he confirms the story."

Here Miss Peters paused, probably for effect, and then dropped her bomb: "Mae, Tommy's mother is planning to charge you with abuse." I looked up in time to catch a glint of satisfaction in those cold gray eyes. The lady had the upper hand, and she was going to use it.

Oh my God, I thought, *now she knows my secret: sometimes, when I'm very angry, I can't help but use my hands to control the kids. Now everyone else will know, and they'll realize I'm not the great foster mother they think I am. In fact, they'll think I'm a fraud.*

"You can be assured," she concluded, "that I will do a proper investigation according to the Department of Children and Youth's manual. The instructions are clear: Whenever there's an accusation of abuse, the first step is to interview everyone involved. The second is to send a formal report to a supervisor. That's exactly what I'll do. Then the case will be out of my hands." She stood up and, without so much as a smile or a good-bye, smoothed her skirt, gathered her papers, and marched toward her car.

The first thing I did was call my friend Terry. We met years ago in a foster parents' orientation just after we separated from our husbands. Neither man chose to support his wife and children, so there was no choice; we had to find work. We didn't have the skills to get office jobs, but we did know how to take care of children. That's how we became foster mothers. Terry and I have been a team ever since. People said we even looked alike with our thickening waistlines, simple clothes, and close-cropped, no-nonsense haircuts.

Years ago we founded an organization called Foster Care Mothers United, FCMU for short. It grew out of training sessions the department provided during a time when people believed foster care could be a solution to the problem of neglected and abused children. Some of the same reform-minded child psychologists and family educators who spoke at those training sessions continue to visit FCMU; they still talk about unconditional caring and child-centered learning. Terry and I led the FCMU for many years. I can't count the number of foster mothers we trained and supported. It was good work. But now I needed that support myself.

"I'm in bad trouble, Terry," I told her as soon as she answered the phone. "Miss Peters came over to tell me I'm being accused of abusing Tommy. She's going to help Tommy's mother pursue the charge through the department. This time she actually has the ammunition to get me. You should have seen her; she was even more arrogant than usual."

"This is serious, Mae. You could lose your foster care contract." Pausing to absorb the information, Terry wondered: "Didn't Tommy's mother physically abuse him?"

"He sometimes hints at it, but there's no clear evidence. We do know he was severely beaten by his father; the man once broke his arm. Tommy's mother certainly knew about the beatings, but she didn't, or couldn't, protect her son. During the past year, however, she's been in recovery, and she's doing much better. None of this matters, though. What's important is that Miss Peters is out to get me."

And then I confessed. "Terry, not everything Miss Peters says is a lie. I do get very angry. There are times when I do yell and scream at the kids. Sometimes I have to physically pull Tommy away from a bad situation. A few weeks ago when he hit Tamika on the head with a soccer ball, I was so furious I held him by the shoulders and shook him until he cried. Tommy's mother also told one of the teachers that I slapped him across the face, but I didn't do that. I would never do that. I'm not mean to the kids. Terry, I hope you believe me. Do you?"

Bless her, Terry said, "I've told you many times how much I admire your work. You do wonders with children. And I know you would never hurt a child. But I'm also worried about you, Mae. Every foster mother I know gets angry at the kids from time to time, but you go further. You argue with the mothers when it isn't even necessary. And I've seen you go out of your way to get services neither the mothers nor the case managers deem necessary. I think you care too much."

"But that caring is my strength," I argued. "I want these kids to learn how to behave and to get everything they need. They're good kids, even if they do cause trouble."

"I don't want you to stop fighting for the kids, Mae, all I want is for you to learn how to protect yourself. Not everybody understands foster care the way we do. Most case managers think we're just glorified baby-sitters. They don't believe we can heal anybody! But I don't want to argue with you, especially when you're being attacked. Just remember that I really do believe in your work. Let's see what Miss Peters actually does. Often she doesn't follow through on her threats. Maybe it will all blow over."

Knowing Terry wanted to end the conversation, I asked a favor: "Let's keep this between the two of us. I feel too ashamed to let others know."

Sleep that night was fitful. *Why am I so alone? Doesn't Terry see that this shouldn't be about protecting me? It should be about good care for children. But she's right, I am too emotionally involved. What makes me think I'm a good foster mother and, of all things, their guardian angel? It's a fantasy, an illusion. I can see that now. Who am I anyhow? Just a middle-aged, poorly educated troublemaker!*

One cold December day, when I was putting Tamika down for a nap, Miss Peters called to say she would come by that afternoon to pick up Tommy and David for the next step in the investigation. My heart dropped. And when the boys returned home and avoided my eyes, I felt hopeless.

But it was a busy time of year, too busy for me to focus very long on one thing. Christmas was on its way, so there were presents to buy, and the house had to be decorated. And, of course, Tommy and David had their usual school problems. Tommy got into a fight with a classmate and literally knocked his tooth out. And Tamika needed to be seen by a neurologist. Meanwhile, the problem with Miss Peters continued to brew, although in a slightly different way. She was now insisting that Tommy be tested for psychological problems and perhaps undergo psychiatric care in a hospital. This got me angry. It was wrong to think of hospitalizing him; in fact, it might be just about fatal. He would do better if they all could have a little more patience with him and with me.

When I tried to talk about this with Miss Peters, she got furious. "What makes you such an expert? This child needs special care, psychiatric care. You can't help him. Don't you know that?"

I tried to explain my position in professional language: "Tommy has already experienced considerable trauma. Hospitalizing him would mean he would have to leave home and adjust to still another environment where he knows no one. That would be yet another trauma. Besides, he doesn't need it. What he needs is to feel safe and to learn how to trust, and that's already happening in my house."

Miss Peters grimaced.

In response, I nearly shouted: "Give me the time I need to work with him. If you get him tested, they'll take him away, and that will be the end of him. This is his last chance!"

Miss Peters slowly, patronizingly, explained, "The department hires psychologists to make those decisions, Mae. For the last time, you're not qualified to decide on what's best for Tommy."

I slumped in my chair and said nothing; there was nothing more to say.

The winter was bad. I brooded over the department's investigation and my shortcomings. Over and over I heard myself worry that I was failing as a foster mother. I was too emotionally involved, and I couldn't do the paperwork. All this worrying meant I wasn't able to pay enough attention to the kids, so they got into more fights. Then, one snowy day, while I was making dinner, I heard David scream in pain. I ran into the living room to see that Tommy had stabbed him in the arm with a pair of scissors. Blood had already begun to soak through his shirt.

David bawled, "He took my shoes and wouldn't give them back."

"You cut up my favorite shirt, you motherfucker," Tommy yelled. "And now I'll be the one who gets punished. You're such a crybaby. Mae will feel sorry for you."

I put pressure on the wound until the bleeding stopped, cleaned up David's arm, applied some antiseptic cream, and held him until he stopped crying. He actually fell asleep, so I laid him down on the couch next to me. Meanwhile Tommy had retreated to the far end of the room, looking as mean and defiant as he could. And I fell into the hole in my stomach. *I should have been watching them. I'm not as quick as I used to be. Maybe I have to give up this whole thing.*

Still, I had to deal with Tommy, so I pulled myself together and demanded that he sit down on the chair across from me. We were quiet for a while, just sitting there looking at each other unhappily, and then, as if a dam had broken, he began to cry. I took him in my arms and sang him a lullaby. We spoke no words, but our sadness was intense.

Reports had to be written, official notification made through appropriate channels. Miss Peters was horrified. And I began to give way to despair.

In the early spring a special delivery letter arrived from the department. It was a copy of Miss Peters's report of her interviews with David, Tommy, and his mother. I read it closely, noting how she had asked the children leading questions and how, even in print, Tommy's mother came across as confused and disoriented. *No one will believe this stuff!*

Soon after, however, I got a letter from an administrator in the department saying a hearing would be held to determine my capacity as a foster care parent. Now there was no stopping the process. I had to act, but couldn't find the energy. I did, however, call the therapist I had seen years ago. I knew I needed help.

Meanwhile, Terry convinced me to set aside my shame and bring the problem to FCMU. And then she led the way. "Don't you realize what's going on here?" she asked the group. "Any of us could be Mae. Any of us could be accused just like she is. Sure she makes mistakes, but she creates a loving home. We know she's helped many kids; in fact, she saved several of them. Remember when little Mary was supposed to go home to her sexually abusive father, and Mae got the department to stop the action? And don't forget that she also supported us when the agency reduced our payment scale. She even testified about it before the city council! We must support her when she needs us!"

The group resolved to write a letter in support of me to the director of the department. They also decided to speak to parents they knew and ask them to write letters. Someone offered to help me write my own report refuting Miss Peters's accusations. And during the week after the meeting, several called to admit that they, too, lost patience and sometimes got physical with their own foster children. They all wanted to help. I was thankful but not very hopeful. And I didn't do anything to help myself. Often I would hear myself say, *You deserve this, Mae. You shouldn't be a foster mother.*

I was beating myself up, and I knew it. But why? In therapy, I remembered my mother's anger, how furious she could be at me, and how it came out when I least expected it, as a slap across my face or a hurtful comment. On the other hand, as soon as my father walked into the house she became weak, and she couldn't protect me from my father's anger. I knew I was doing much better than she had done—but not well enough. Tommy was a test. But would I pass it?

My therapist kept saying the challenge was to stop beating myself up and, instead, to find a way to love myself. When I told her I was at a loss to figure out how to do that, she smiled and said, "I know it's hard. But it's possible. Let's try."

We actually meditated together. She asked me to silently repeat the words *You deserve this, Mae. You shouldn't be a foster mother,* and then to scan my body for sensations. That was easy. I was used to the lump in my throat and the tears that came when I beat myself up. But when I started crying, I couldn't stop. And the words *You deserve this, Mae,* kept blaring in my head.

I had the image of a river of tears that started flowing when I was a kid. And I remembered past hurts that only made me cry more. It seemed the tears and the memories would never stop. At one point I think I must have gotten scared, because I wanted to stop meditating. But Barbara suggested that I try to continue, if at all possible. And so I did—until my hour was almost over. Then a funny thing happened. I suddenly saw myself in a boat paddling down my own river of tears—and I had the three kids with me! Amazingly, they looked happy. David was proudly showing me a fish that was bigger than he was. The image made me laugh. And I said aloud, *Maybe I'm not so bad after all.*

Unfortunately, this state of mind didn't last for long. Soon I was back to my old internal harangue—*You don't fool yourself. You know you're a fraud no matter what Barbara says.*

Finally, a letter came informing me of a hearing date. It would take place in the grand old courthouse that now housed the main office of the city's Department of Children and Youth, on Monday, April 15th, just three weeks away. When that day came, I climbed the three banks of steps toward the large pair of bronze doors, burdened by my heavy winter coat and my fear. Inside, the meeting room was bland, with gray walls and white window shades. Miss Peters and Tommy's mother sat on one side of a long, bare table, silent and angry. I took a seat on the other side and waited in silence for what seemed like hours until the administrator entered and seated himself at the head of the table. A heavyset man with owlish eyes behind thick glasses, he blew his nose with a great deal of noise before opening the thin manila folder he brought with him. I quickly realized it contained nothing but a blank writing pad, the petition, and Miss Peters's report.

When asked about my performance, Miss Peters replied: "Mae is a very difficult person to supervise. She almost never gets her monthly reports in on time, and when confronted, she has a hostile attitude. I have tried to point this out to her, but it hasn't helped. Nor is she cooperating on the issue of getting expert care for Tommy, one of the children housed with her. And we have evidence that she uses corporal punishment to discipline him."

Tommy's mother added, "My son told me she abuses him, and I know he's telling the truth."

Abuses him—that is a lie! But the administrator isn't challenging it.

Besides, they're confusing my paperwork with my performance as a foster mother. He isn't challenging that either. And no one is mentioning the good work I've done with children over the past twenty-one years. How can they do this to me?

When my turn came, I argued that the accusation of abuse was exaggerated. I claimed the testimony of the children was taken under intimidating circumstances, because they were afraid of the very person who was interviewing them, namely, Miss Peters. I also said the accusations regarding my administrative work were irrelevant to the charge of abuse and should not be considered. But I was a wimp. There was no heart to my little speech. I couldn't muster the energy to fight for myself. The supervisor duly took his notes and said little.

As he pulled the meeting to a close, I asked about the next steps in the process. In response, he looked straight at me, and I saw his inert lifeless eyes for the first time. That's when I knew he really didn't care what happened to Tommy or me. But he did carefully mouth the words, "We are all very concerned with bringing this case to closure, and be assured, you will receive a letter from the department in due time."

A month later I got that letter. It said that as of June 30th of that year, my foster care contract with the department would be terminated. It was a form letter. There was no expression of concern for me or the kids, no consideration for the effect it would have on our lives. However, the letter did include a section on how to initiate the departmental appeal process.

A few weeks later, Tommy was transferred to a residential setting for more disturbed children in order to be evaluated for further treatment. Poor kid; he didn't want to go in the worst way. When Miss Peters told him, he screamed at her and smashed several of his favorite toys, including his precious Game Boy. And he cried uncontrollably when she came to pick him up.

Tommy's transfer came as a real blow. I knew I hadn't fought well for either of us, but it was the department's mismanagement of his case that I couldn't get out of my mind. I watched the angry thoughts swirl through my mind: *It's wrong, cruel, to pluck him out of a family he wants to be in.*

Nobody ever asked him whether he wanted to move or what he needed to feel better, just as nobody paid any attention to me or my view of Tommy's problems. The department's arbitrary actions have to be challenged—and I'm angry enough to do it! Tommy doesn't deserve such treatment!

It's hard to believe, but I actually stopped brooding and began taking action to protect him. I also found the courage to fight for myself. Terry applauded when she heard about it. "I knew you had it in you!"

I also visited Tommy. Seeing me, he jumped into my arms and wouldn't let go: "I don't like it here, Mae," he cried. "Please take me back to your house. I'm afraid of the bigger boys. See that one, the boy in the red shirt? He punches me in the stomach whenever we're alone. Mae, I miss you and David and Tamika. Please take me away. Please!"

My heart went out to him. I wished I could take him home, but I knew that was just about impossible. However, I said I would try. All I could do was to try. Most important, I had to keep him out of a psychiatric hospital. So I got busy looking for people who could help. A member of the city council got interested, as did a local community group. One contact led to another, and a lawyer volunteered. I told them and anyone else who would listen, "This boy doesn't need to take the institutional route."

"I can't believe you're doing this," Terry said when we talked on the telephone. "Tommy's mother is attacking you, the boy isn't even in your house anymore, and you're still fighting—and against people who can take away your contract. Mae, you're asking for more trouble!"

"Do you really want me to give up on that boy, Terry? That's just what the department wants! It would be a lot worse than grabbing him by the shoulders and shaking him. Don't you see that what they're doing is wrong? Tommy is not a throwaway child! I'm going to resist his hospitalization no matter what the department does. If I give in after all of this, I'll never forgive myself."

And then, about a month later, I visited Tommy again. It was a visit I would never forget. Much to my surprise, he was a happier child. The director of the program held his hand as we said hello, and he looked up at her adoringly. Tommy had found another mother-figure to love him. And when I watched him play, I could see he was one of the boys. He had found another home. I must admit to feeling hurt, almost betrayed. It seemed I cared more than he did. Something was wrong, and it was inside me.

After the visit I felt a little foolish. I wasn't as important as I thought. And I didn't feel quite as indignant about the department. It's not that I thought Tommy's case was being managed well, but I wasn't as exasperated and panicked. Others were there to help him, too; his well-being didn't depend entirely on me. Actually, the change in my feelings worried me; I wondered if I would be less effective as an advocate for Tommy. As it turned out, the opposite was true.

In therapy, I raged and complained about Miss Peters and the department until I was tired of hearing myself. The anger was in my dreams, in my relationship to my foster kids, all over the place. And inside I was terribly hurt—much like the unloved child I had been in the past. One day, when I was yelling at David, I caught a glimpse of my angry face in the mirror. It was contorted and blustery, rather ugly. The irony is that the kids hadn't done anything to make me that angry. The whole scene felt so absurd that I started to laugh. Was I yelling at *them*? At my *parents*? Maybe I was yelling at *myself*. But why? The kids were confused by my laughter, but when I reached out to them, they came into my arms. Soon we were all rolling on the floor, giggling with the silliness of it all. And I felt such a tremendous surge of compassion for them—and me— it was as if my heart had burst. I was freeing myself . . . slowly.

Meanwhile, the appeal process on my case slowly worked its way through the departmental system. Special delivery letters arrived, the next phase of the appeal process was announced, and still more meetings were held. I was more skillful than I had been at first. I asked the parents of other foster care children I had taken care of to help, and many of them wrote letters or spoke to people they knew in the department. I sought the help of a lawyer who researched the current laws on contractual relationships to clarify my rights. And my friends were behind me.

Finally, I got another letter informing me of the date of the appeal hearing. It would take place before a senior administrator in the same old courthouse. In preparation, I personally sent him a copy of my own report on the incident with Tommy and made sure he had copies of all the letters that had been sent in my defense. On the appointed day I climbed those same marble steps and sat in that same somber hearing room. This time the administrator was dressed informally; no jacket, rolled-up shirt sleeves, and an open collar. His warm brown eyes and broad smile seemed to say, "Be at ease with me. I won't hurt you." I knew enough to be wary. The hearing might be taking place in a court building, but it wasn't a court of law. This wasn't a trial but an administrative process, and that meant it wasn't necessarily fair or objective. There were no legal statutes to protect me; in fact, I was told I couldn't even bring in my own lawyer!

Sure enough, after the administrator's first few words, I sensed trouble. He seemed to have all the materials I had sent, but his examples relied almost entirely on Miss Peters's report. "I see here," he began in a reserved tone, "that you don't get your reports in on time and that you often question your supervisor's authority. You have to understand, this organization relies on its supervisory staff, so we must support them. And that means foster care parents must support them as well. That includes getting the paperwork done on time, Mae. And let's not forget your behavior with Tommy. Using your hands to discipline children cannot be tolerated."

Feeling my throat constrict, I swallowed hard, straightened my back, and argued my defense coolly—at least he was giving me that opportunity. I talked calmly about my work with Tommy, his help with chores, his tears when I visited him at his new site, the trusting relationship we had developed, and his impulsive violence. I argued that he had improved and would continue to, if not subjected to the trauma of hospitalization. And I offered to give him another try in my house, especially if I could work with a psychologist to give him the limits he needed at home.

To my surprise, the administrator seemed to appreciate what I was saying. I became a little hopeful. *This is my chance to talk about the bigger issues*, I thought to myself. *I can give him a view of the foster care system as only a foster mother knows it.*

And so I began. "With all due respect, I would like to take a few moments of your time to talk about how decisions about children are made in the department." When the administrator nodded his approval, I continued, "Unfortunately, neither foster care parents nor their foster children are included in rulings that will change their lives . . . "

He seemed genuinely interested in what I had to say, and he wanted to know more about FMCU—particularly the organization's effort to give the foster parents more of a role in assessing the needs of children. I felt encouraged.

By the time the meeting ended, I knew I had handled myself well. I hadn't undercut my case by exploding with anger, nor had I become a wimp. But this alone wasn't enough to save my job. Whichever way it went, however, I knew the decision wouldn't destroy me. I had learned something about the love that was under my anger. And by now I was a rather good advocate. Even if, in the end, I lost the right to care for foster children directly, I would continue to advocate for their rights—and for the rights of their caregivers. While this felt good to say to myself, I also knew that if I wasn't reinstated, the advocacy would be tough to do as a "disgraced" former foster mother.

That very night I had a dream that woke me up. In this dream, all of us—Tommy, David, Terry, Miss Peters, and the department administrator—were in a bus together. It was dark and dangerous outside, and the bus was going too fast for the road. Somehow I understood that nobody knew where we were going. And I was frightened. Actually, everyone was frightened. At the moment I woke up, my feelings shifted, and I felt terribly sad and so protective of everyone that my heart ached.

A month later a report of the department's findings came in the mail. In the midst of the many negative comments about my behavior, there was a brief sentence indicating that I would be allowed to continue my work with foster children. David and Tamika could continue to live with me. They would not cancel my contracts.

From another source within the department, I also learned that Tommy would not be sent to a psychiatric hospital. I felt jubilant, absolved.

You did it, Mae, I said to myself. *You fought for Tommy, you fought for yourself . . . and you won! Not only that, you also worked with your anger and found love and compassion. Whoever said you were a fraud?*

"What is to give light must endure burning."

—VIKTOR FRANKS

ANGER AND COMPASSION

There's an old tale about a young girl, perhaps nine or ten, who was walking along the beach one morning when she came upon hundreds of starfish that had been marooned on the sand during a storm. Looking closely, she saw that many of them were still struggling to stay alive. So she picked up one after another of these helpless beings and threw them as far out into the water as she could.

A man who was also walking along the beach watched her for a little while and then called out above the roar of the ocean, "Why are you wasting your time throwing a few starfish back into the water? Don't you see there are hundreds of them? It's a waste of time. Your effort won't make any difference."

In response, the little girl picked up another starfish, threw it into the water, and called back, "It will make a difference to that one!"

What is the value of a single starfish? It doesn't serve any function for people and therefore has no monetary value. You can't trade it for anything, so it has no exchange value. Just like the man in the story, most of us would barely notice a single starfish's existence, let alone try to save it. But this little girl was different. In her eyes, each starfish had value simply because it was alive. Their distress kindled her compassion, and so she saved as many as she could. Because it felt good, the effort became a gift that she gave to herself.

Similarly, Mae sensed the value in one small, very troubled boy named Tommy. People asked, "Why are you trying so hard? You can't do it all. Besides, the department will take care of him." Her answer, often difficult for her to express, was that Tommy *mattered*. She had to help him. Besides, helping was essential to who she was.[1]

Compassion is one of life's most remarkable gifts. With it, we are part of the ongoing work of creation. By nurturing and protecting other living beings, not only do we help others, but in doing so we ourselves thrive. On the other hand, if we don't take part in the work of creation, we feel isolated and alone.

Compassion is grounded in the reality of *interbeing*. Thich Nhat Hanh, who introduced this word, uses it to indicate that in this world we do, indeed, live in and through each other. Green plants and human beings inter-are because we're composed of the same basic chemicals, and we rely on the same sunlight and the same water. All living beings emerge, manifest, and then die. And so the giant redwood threatened by a chainsaw can generate our compassion. At a very basic level, we are one.[2]

The same was true of Mae and Tommy. Both felt the pain of loneliness; both ached for some human nurturing. Mae sensed it in Tommy, and there's reason to believe Tommy sensed it in Mae. He cared about her. As compassion flowed between them, they both thrived.

At times Mae's compassion turned into exceptionally skillful parenting. For instance, when David said the pirates told him to take Tamika's toy, she didn't reject him or call his story a lie; instead, she joined in the fantasy, sensing that this, too, was a way children learn. And when Tommy belligerently scowled at her after hurting David, Mae made room for his pain by holding him in her angry-compassionate gaze. In response, Tommy gave up his belligerence and broke into tears, which meant she could nurture him with a hug. Mae's anger-compassion was a fire that kept her and the children warm.

Unfortunately, anger often overpowered her compassion—and that was deeply upsetting to her. Indeed, for many years she hid her anger, even from herself. Sometimes, especially when she presented herself to others as the children's guardian angel, she suspected she was a fraud. This was a big price to pay for the false comfort that denial brings.

In psychotherapy, Mae was eventually able to recognize that at times she was an angry person. But she still found many ways to blame her anger on others. When she took the step of accepting the reality, the *isness*, of her anger, there was no longer any point in arguing about it. As with any other emotion, her anger just was. What she could do was to increase her awareness of it; she could deconstruct it—and see what other emotions were involved.

In so doing, she remembered how anger was used in her family, in particular how her mother was a terror with the children and a wimp with her husband. Mae became aware that her own anger was often flavored by fear and shame. Sometimes these flavors increased the intensity of her anger, and she exploded in rage. In front of an authority, however, they did the opposite, and, as a result, she felt helpless. She, too, was either a terror or a wimp.

And one day, after the boys broke her favorite lamp, she felt her fingers grow tight as they forged themselves into weapons that could grab and shake them. It was a deeply upsetting experience for Mae. When she talked about it in my office, I asked her to close her eyes and focus her awareness on the upset she felt in her body. She talked about the urge to run out of the office and hide—and she named the feeling "humiliation." It was hard for her to keep focused on that difficult feeling, but she did so until it faded. Several hours after our session, she called to say that she continued to feel lots of inner turmoil after the session, but most recently compassion for herself bubbled up. She asked, "Do you think my compassion is real or just another of my attempts to escape responsibility?"

"If the feeling exists, it's real," I responded. "Your challenge is to accept the is-ness of all these feelings—the anger, the humiliation, *and* the compassion. In fact, you need to hold the complexity of those feelings in your two hands and be true to the blend."

In meditation Mae took still another important step: she knew her anger as a kind of energy. She felt it move through her as a kind of "push" or "potency." It could motivate action.

We all experience this energy. Can you remember a time when someone stepped on your toes? Perhaps you were aware of the feeling of anger rising inside you, much like a surge of heat. That's anger-energy. Can you remember being on a high-speed roadway when a car swerved into your lane? Did the muscles in your body tighten in an attempt to protect you? That, too, is anger-energy. Anger is a fact of nature, a flow of vitality that surges in response to perceived danger.

In this sense, anger, like any other emotion, is similar to water: it is fluid and changeable. It can take on the hue of fear, compassion, or other emotions. It can move through the body and the mind rather rapidly or freeze and stay for a long time. It can also move between people. Have you ever noticed how a nasty comment begets other nasty comments, how a smile begets other smiles? As emotions move, they have impact. Sometimes it seems as if this impact is simply internal, and that you are the only one in your family or workplace feeling angry or sad or happy. But emotions spread among people, even if they aren't aware of it.

And sometimes, when the energy of anger within a group builds upon itself, people use it collectively, perhaps to suppress the freedom of others or to make war. We have many examples of that in world history. The same is true of compassion. Because we inter-are, one person's compassion can build on another's and have an effect on a family or a neighborhood. A single act of compassion can build on other compassionate acts to alter a child's entire life. Sometimes anger tempered by compassion can be the input that builds on other inputs to alter the foster care system of an entire city. By no means is this a strange idea. Public relations people, advertising firms, and spin doctors all bank on this multiplier phenomenon. They know that the timely placement of an advertisement, the right phrase spoken in the right venue, and the correct spin on an event can all build on each other and ultimately create the desired outcome.

Under the right conditions and given the caprice of probability, people in combination with others of like mind can trigger a series of reactions that ultimately changes the world—perhaps for the good of all rather than for a particular political or commercial interest.

There's a story from the world of science that might help shed light on how this happens. The story is about Edward Lorenz, a weatherman who wanted to do a better job of accurately predicting the weather. He began his research by asking whether it was even possible. Up until the middle of the twentieth century, there was little doubt that the answer to that question was *yes*. Most people accepted Isaac Newton's premise that our entire world was rule-bound, and that weather systems were as predictable as the rotation of the planets. It was believed that all we needed to accurately predict the weather was the right method. With the aid of a computer, Lorenz found a way to test that hypothesis.

Lorenz ran the thousands upon thousands of calculations needed to determine whether Newton was right. And in 1979, he wrote a paper entitled "Predictability: Does the Flap of a Butterfly's Wings in Brazil Set Off a Tornado in Texas?" In this paper, he answered his butterfly question with a *yes* that negated Newton's hypothesis and proved that the weather is essentially unpredictable.

Lorenz's research demonstrated that tiny differences in "input," such as the flap of a butterfly's wings, could result in overwhelming differences in "output." In other words, minor fluctuations in local weather conditions could build on each other to cause major shifts that affect the vast weather systems blanketing our globe. A flap of a butterfly's wings in Brazil could be the genesis of a storm system in Texas at a later time. However, Lorenz added, because there are so *many* minor fluctuations, with such a wide range of effects on local conditions, weather is not fully predictable—and never will be.

This research has proven that pattern emerges within the chaos of weather systems, predictable or not. In fact, scientists can track how patterns emerge and become elaborated. The phenomenon has acquired a technical name: *sensitive dependence on initial conditions*. Half jokingly, however, scientists continue to call it the Butterfly Effect.[3]

Extrapolating from this research, we can say there's a relationship between the frequency of angry actions and the amount of suffering in the world. We can also say there's a relationship between the frequency of compassionate acts and the degree of well-being in the world. It also follows that an act of anger tempered by compassion is a force that can tilt our civilization toward protecting and nurturing all living beings. In this sense, Mae's effort to help Tommy is changing the world.

In the following meditation we'll work with anger. However, if you feel this is inappropriate for you at this time, or if some other emotion is more important, you can change the meditation to suit your need. The work will be essentially the same, though the content will be different.

Please remember that all emotions are composed of thoughts in the mind, feelings in the body, and sometimes images that occur when your eyes are closed. Indeed, our work in this meditation will include deconstructing anger into bodily sensations, internal images, and internal talk.

In previous meditations, the intent was to learn how to saturate each of these sense gates with awareness so that the experience, whatever it was, would reemerge as richly and as fully as possible in the present. We have practiced this method without *intentionally* accessing a particular emotion. In this meditation, that practice will change; now we'll *intentionally* access an emotion—anger—in the form of an angry memory. And then we'll explore the memory at the sense gate(s) where it is most fully experienced.

To be successful, this meditation needs to be tailored to fit your own needs. For some of us, body sensations are easiest to access. For others, internal images or internal talk are easier to access. Given that, you will need to decide which sense gate(s) best express your angry emotion. Please don't assume you know already—each meditation offers another opportunity to discover something about yourself. And as Shinzen often says, "Subtle is significant." A hint of sadness can add another dimension to anger, a fleeting image can cast a new light on your anger's impermanence, a jumble of words can lead to insight.

Please remember, especially if meditating on emotions is a fairly new effort for you, that this skill takes considerable time to learn. Meditation is a 2,500-year-old science of the mind; it cannot be learned from one meditation or one book. My hope is that experimenting with the meditations in this book will tempt you to search for a teacher or a sitting group and so enrich your practice. And now, on to the meditation.

Before beginning, give yourself permission to recall a moment when you felt angry. Choose a recent experience. And give yourself the freedom to make a meaningful choice. Perhaps you'll remember the feeling of annoyance rather than anger. Maybe it will be rage. This doesn't matter; they're all angry emotions. And if nothing comes up, let the request sit in the back of your mind as a question you're seeking to answer. You might hear an answer in a few minutes, an hour, or a week.

Alternatively, you may have several experiences of anger in mind and not know which to settle on. Let yourself decide on one, remembering that if it doesn't work, you're always free to choose another—in another try at the meditation.

You might choose an entirely different emotion, substituting it for anger. Perhaps it will be an emotion associated with the trouble you've been working with during these meditations. In the end there is no "right" choice; everything is a grist for the mill. Once you've chosen a memory, you're ready for the meditation that follows.

One by one, you will access each of the sense gates we're working with: sensations in the body, internal images, and internal talk. By feeling, watching, and listening, you'll deconstruct these different components of your angry emotion. Then, with greater specificity, you'll begin to put the entire emotion back together again. This is the way of Mindfulness Meditation.

Once again, review the entire meditation first, then read and do it section by section. Once you learn the meditation, you won't need this cumbersome procedure. Also keep your journal close at hand—and don't forget the timer.

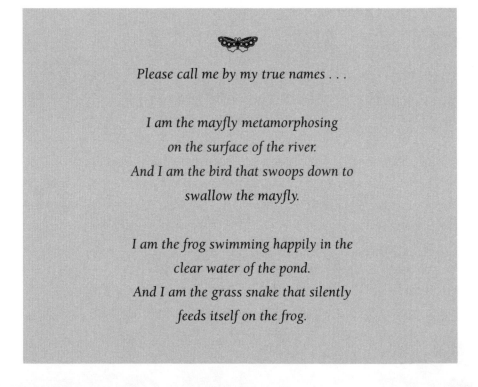

Please call me by my true names . . .

I am the mayfly metamorphosing
on the surface of the river.
And I am the bird that swoops down to
swallow the mayfly.

I am the frog swimming happily in the
clear water of the pond.
And I am the grass snake that silently
feeds itself on the frog.

I am the child in Uganda, all skin and bones,
my legs as thin as bamboo sticks.
And I am the arms merchant selling
deadly weapons to Uganda.

I am the twelve-year-old girl, refugee on a
small boat who throws herself into the
ocean after being raped by a sea pirate.
And I am the pirate, my heart not yet
capable of seeing and loving . . .

Please call me by my true names so I can
wake up and the door of my heart could
be left open, the door of compassion.

—THICH NHAT HANH

A Meditation on Anger

Settle into a meditative position with your back straight, your stomach muscles relaxed, and your head inclined slightly forward. Close your eyes and relax into your body. As you breathe, let a small smile spread across your face. Hundreds of small muscles will loosen as you do so. Take a moment to feel the body sensation of relaxation.

Now, on to your angry memory. Recall the person . . . the group . . . that was involved. Imagine what happened . . . the place where it occurred. And please feel free to substitute another emotion, perhaps one that's triggered by the trouble you have been working on in these meditations.

*Then shift some of your awareness to the body, and scan those places in the body where feelings tend to occur . . . in the face . . . neck . . . shoulders . . . and trunk. Wait for any **body sensation** that arises.*

Perhaps the sensations that arise feel more like fear than anger . . . more like sadness than anger. That's fine. This is material to work with in the future. Label the location in your body.

You might sense a tightness in the throat or a constriction in your chest that signals anger. Maybe the emotion will take the form of a headache. Be curious, and label the location in your body. Just feel.

Pay special attention if the body sensation changes. What was a tightness in your throat may become tears in your eyes. What was a headache might become a flutter in your abdomen. Label the location and feel the impermanence.

Perhaps the angry memory will fade . . . or the body sensation that came with it will disappear. Try to find it again. If it doesn't appear, this may be a time to end.

Take five minutes to do this phase of the meditation . . . and end it at a point when the body sensation fades or when it changes, even subtly.

❀

*Again, begin with the angry memory, and place your awareness on the screen in front of your closed eyes. Watch . . . and be ready for the arising of an **internal image**.*

Perhaps you will see some kind of likeness . . . an outline of a person . . . thing . . . or place associated with the angry memory. Perhaps an image arises that seems to have nothing to do with it. Whichever, label it clear.

Maybe you will see a fuzzy suggestion of an image . . . something fleeting and barely present . . . related or unrelated to your memory. Label that subtle.

With the memory of your anger in mind, watch the arising and fading of images in front of your eyes.

If no clear or subtle image arises, label it none, *and rest in the flow of colors . . . or in the shifting light that comes through your eyelids.*

Take five minutes to do this phase of the meditation.

❀

*Now place your awareness in the place where **internal talk** takes place. Perhaps it's in your ear canals, perhaps it's between your two ears and toward the back of your head.*

Recall the memory of your anger . . . and listen. You may catch internal talk well after it has come and gone. That doesn't matter . . . simply be aware.

Perhaps your internal talk comes in words that are well defined. Whether they are about your memory or something entirely different, label them clear. *Just listen.*

Or, what you hear may be disorganized . . . barely audible . . . or an almost undetectable sound that may or may not be connected to your memory. Whichever, label that subtle.

Then again, you may hear nothing at all. If that's so, label that none *and sit in the silence. There is no right way.*

Please be patient with yourself . . . accept what is . . . listen and wait.

Take five minutes to continue this phase of the meditation.

✦

Now, recall the angry memory and turn to the **body sensation** *that comes with it. If the feeling is gone, imagine it. Then place some of your awareness on the screen in front of your eyes and wait for an* **internal image** *associated with your anger. If no image arises, simply keep some of your awareness on the screen and some on a body sensation you associate with anger.*

With the memory of your anger, keep some of your awareness on the screen in front of your eyes and watch for an **internal image.** *Keep some of your awareness in your two ear canals and listen for* **internal talk.**

Last, with the memory of your anger, keep some of your awareness in your two ear canals and listen for **internal talk.** *Also keep some of your awareness on* **body sensations.**

Now . . . set your timer for ten minutes, recall the emotional memory, and go through the different dyads—body–image . . . image–talk . . . talk–body.

✦

When the ten minutes are over . . . recall the angry memory one last time. Feel it in your body . . . see it on the screen in front of your eyes . . . and hear it as internal talk. This is a complete experience of your anger . . . Body-Image-Talk.

Take five minutes to continue this meditation

✦

Now . . . slowly open your eyes. Take notes on your experience, if you like. And congratulate yourself for exercising your meditative muscle.

As you no doubt know, this exercise is not an easy challenge. It takes a lot of practice to meditate on anger skillfully.

However, simply making the effort is important. Trying takes courage and strength of will—and puts you on a path toward a fuller . . . more inclusive . . . awareness of the nature of self. This is a path toward wholeness.

May all beings know wholeness.

Training for Awareness

1. Recall your angry memory and scan the body for any sensations. Label locations.

2. Recall your angry memory and watch for any internal images. Label *clear, subtle,* or *none.*

3. Recall your angry memory and listen for any internal talk. Label *clear, subtle,* or *none.*

4. Recall your angry memory and move from body–image to image–talk to talk–body—two sense gates at once.

5. Recall your angry memory and experience it as body–image–talk—three sense gates at one time.

Eight

Harriet's Love Story

I can still remember that moment when I was sorting the mail in our kitchen and noticed an envelope postmarked Savannah, Georgia. I knew immediately it was from Ron, but I tucked it into the pocket of my bathrobe because my husband was nearby. Simply touching the paper made the ground move an inch or two. Not that the letter could change anything. The hard fact was that Ron and I were married to different people. Besides, I was ten pounds overweight, and the wrinkles on my face were getting deeper each day.

Still, my friends thought I was beautiful, an earth figure. There were moments, they said, when they caught a glimpse of the radiant African queen I was meant to be. Somewhere inside I knew what they meant; there was something special in me, if I could only let it out. Instead, I hid myself in large flowing caftans, and all I could think about were dinner menus, shopping lists, and reruns of old lost arguments with my husband, Fred. My house was a mess. The magazines, coffee mugs, and assorted papers that covered most of the surfaces announced my lethargy. Something was wrong.

At age fifty-eight, I was the mother of four, the grandmother of two, a retired teacher, and a member of the local school board. I ought to have been pleased with my life, but I wasn't. Neither was Fred. A tall, angular man whose parents were born in Norway, he rarely spoke, although if you tapped into his mind you might hear a brilliant strategy for winning the next battle at the bank where he worked. I knew he felt hurt and unloved inside, the victim of forces he couldn't control, but on the outside he was cold and aloof.

That evening as I looked at him across the dinner table, I tried to read his almost impenetrable face for the signals of danger, be it a lackluster flatness in his eyes, tightness around his mouth, or a sharper angle to his jaw. This time I had no doubt; he was angry, and it could be directed toward me at any time.

"Did we get the bill from the plumber?" he asked between spoonfuls of the split pea soup I had made.

At least he was talking to me. It wouldn't be another one of those silent dinners. But I had to be careful; the subject of money could be very dangerous. "Yes, it came yesterday. I haven't opened it yet to see what he charged."

"Just like you to put it off," he grumbled. "Don't you know how tight we are?"

I raised my eyes just in time to catch an angry flicker across his. And my stomach tightened. "Fred, please don't pick a fight. You know we planned for this expense."

"You're avoiding the problem. Why can't you remember that my income has gone down over the past six months?"

Then the disdain. "You're doing that sidestep shuffle again, trying to hide the facts from me one more time."

I said nothing. It was better to absorb the insult; that way, he might just let me be. Fred was always finding something wrong. If it wasn't about money, it was the spread of my hips or the way I kissed. How I hoped he wouldn't want sex tonight. Another round of his get-it-up, pump-away, and fall-asleep routine would be more than I could bear.

Then an image of Ron as I once knew him, a beautiful dark brown adolescent boy, flashed across my mind. The memory was so sweet, sweet and tender. My first love.

Fred finally moved into the living room and settled down to watch the news. I washed the dishes and, slowly so as not to arouse his interest, walked upstairs, went into the bathroom, and locked the door. I ran my fingers across the words on the envelope, trying to imagine Ron writing them, then quickly tore it open.

> *Dear Harriet,*
>
> *I know you must be very surprised to hear from me. It's been such a long time since we've been in touch—thirty-one years and five months, to be exact. As you can see from the invitation I've included, our high school class is having a reunion next June. I'm planning to go. Would you consider taking a plane down to join me?*
>
> *I often think of you and those magical days we spent together. Perhaps it's not too late to renew our friendship.*
>
> *I hope you, Fred, and the kids are doing well.*
>
> *Forever,*
> *Ron*

Whenever I thought about that man, I felt blessed. Just to have known him was enough. Such a good man. He even found a way to say hello to my whole family by mentioning Fred and the kids. I wondered what life would have been like if I had married him.

The letter got me thinking about my past and the awful events that led to our first meeting. For me, it all started in Detroit, 1942, when I was about six years old and my life fell apart. My father was fighting in North Africa while my mother and I were trying to survive in a small apartment. I can't remember much about that apartment except that I knew it wasn't home.

Those were bleak times. My mother missed my father badly. Nothing held her interest except our daily walk around the neighborhood to count the number of gold and silver stars hanging in the windows. Silver was for a son or a husband who was wounded in action; gold meant he was dead. My mother cried whenever a new star was added.

Then came the day when we received the telegram and hung up our own gold star. I can still feel a shiver go through me as I think of it. My mother got into bed and didn't get up. And she didn't talk sense. I remember pleading with her, "Wake up, Mama, let's go for a walk. Get up, Mama, do you want something to eat?"

Nothing seemed to get through. Finally, one night while I was asleep, she walked straight out into the street naked as can be, screaming hysterically for my father. I didn't find out about it until the next morning, when a neighbor told me the police had taken her away and put her in a hospital. I can't remember much more, except that I didn't cry. I've always wondered why.

Anyway, I stayed with our neighbor friends for a while. They were kind, elderly people but too sick to take care of me, so I was put on a bus and sent to Savannah, Georgia, where my mother's parents lived. You can probably imagine how frightened I was, never having met my grandparents or been to Georgia. My mother never talked about her family except to say I wasn't missing anything. As it turned out, Savannah was the best thing that ever happened to me—it was a dream come true. I was finally where I belonged. I was home.

Ron was the boy who lived next door. I think I loved him from the first time we met. "Some people are born special," my grandmother would say, "and Ron is one of them." There was nothing he couldn't do: fix a fence, build a birdhouse, catch a bat, or run like there was no tomorrow.

On the very day I arrived he came over and introduced himself. "Hello," he said, fumbling with the bag of early June peas he had picked for me. "I'm Ron, and I'll be your friend, if you want." We took a walk around the neighborhood that afternoon, and he told me about the angry old woman who lived across the street and the man who gave out sweets any time you visited his house. There were more kids on that block than I ever knew in Detroit. Rob and I weren't in the same class at school, but he would always say hello as we passed in the hall, and often we ate lunch together. He even protected me from the bully who lived on the next block.

I remember as clearly as if it were yesterday the moment when he became more than a friend. It was the first time we took a grown-up walk together. I was twelve and he was fourteen. The summer air was moist. Our bodies were hot. When we reached the outskirts of town, he put his arms around me, and I felt him shiver. That made me so embarrassed I started to giggle. But before I could say anything, he reached over and kissed me on the lips. His dark brown eyes flashed in the sunlight, and I felt my face grow hot. We embraced while my heart beat wildly, and then, hand in hand, laughing all the way, we ran as fast as we could to the local soda fountain, where we bought chocolate ice cream sodas.

What wonderful times we had! We did our homework together, delivered papers, and explored the far reaches of town on bikes. I became very courageous, even outrageous, a part of me I lost in future years. Once I even managed to get invited on a vacation to the shore with Ron's family. Granted, it was easy because his parents always said yes, but still, I was a young girl who wasn't used to asserting herself. Of course, our relationship was very innocent. We never did anything more than kiss and hold hands. It was a charmed life. And someone else was taking care of my mother. I was naive enough to think it would last forever.

Then one morning my grandparents received a letter saying my mother had been released from the hospital and was coming to visit. They read it and got angry. She was trouble, they said. I always knew there was something wrong between them, but I didn't know how bad it was. The small cloud that had hovered in the distance of my life grew ominous.

"Your mother was born bad," my grandmother said, "like a bad seed." To her way of thinking, they offered her a good life but she couldn't appreciate it. My grandfather was a successful real estate agent in Savannah, so they lived well. My mother was their only child and it seems she got almost anything she wanted.

Still, my mother certainly wasn't happy. She smoked and dated the wrong kind of boys. She even tried to run away a few times. Then she got pregnant and had to have an abortion. Worst of all, a few years later she married my father—an unskilled wanderer my grandparents called white trash. They never forgave her.

So my mother's letter was not welcome. But I didn't pay too much attention to their feelings; once I knew my mother was coming, I discovered a hollow ache inside me. I wanted her again, whoever she was.

I was sitting at the kitchen table doing my homework when she arrived. I looked out the window in time to see her walking toward the house and ran out to greet her. She dropped her bags and hugged me tightly, too tightly, crying all the time. I stood very still while she traced my face with her forefingers, as if she was trying to learn me once again. But her words were meant for a six-year-old.

"Baby doll, you're so cute," she said, playing with my curls. "Are you being a good girl for Grandma and Grandpa? We're going to have such a good time together, you and I. Remember how you liked me to read storybooks to you? We'll do it again."

As she settled in, she acted as if I were still a little girl that she could bring up. I took it as an insult. Sure, she missed the chance to raise me, but why couldn't she understand it was too late? Besides, she was bossy. She didn't like Ron, thought I didn't dress warmly enough, and insisted I eat whatever was served. We fought every day.

Worse still, she decided to settle us in New York. That meant I had to leave everyone I loved, including Ron. The two of us were inconsolable. How we cried! How we begged! But nothing we said mattered. Still, we were determined not to let my mother get between us. I remember the night before I left as if it were yesterday. The scent of peonies filled the early spring air. We sat on the back porch and held each other, vowing that our love would last forever. In our hearts, we remained true to that vow.

The next morning my mother and I boarded a train headed for the Bronx. I hated that place even before I saw it, and as the days passed my hatred only increased. Our apartment was small, and there was no grass to play on, no trees to swing from, and no friends. We fought more than ever. But Ron stayed in my heart like a bright red ruby. No one could take him from me.

When he wrote and said his family had decided to visit some relatives in New York, I was ecstatic. It was as if I had a reprieve. How I looked forward to that visit! The plan was that we would meet in front of Macy's Department Store at two in the afternoon on August 5. My mother didn't approve but didn't try to stop me, probably because she knew it was impossible.

When the day came, I put on my new lavender and green dress, took the subway down to Thirty-fourth Street at noon, and waited for him. I scanned every face, walked up and down the street, and then I waited some more. But there was no Ron. It was well after closing time when I finally gave up and took the subway back to the Bronx, crying all the way.

A week later, I learned he had been waiting at another entrance. Neither of us knew that Macy's was big enough to have entrances on two major avenues. I feared the odds against us were too great.

However, we continued to write. And then, quite suddenly, his letters stopped. At first I was upset; I didn't know why he would do such a thing. But somewhere inside I began to accept it. We lived too far apart. It wasn't working. My mother kept saying he probably had met someone else and I should forget him. Besides, she kept reminding me that I was too young for such entanglements. Feeling hopeless, half believing her, I, too, eventually stopped writing. How could I have put so much stock in an impossible dream? Soon I was to realize that I was underestimating Ron—and my mother.

One night a few months later, while I was washing the dinner dishes, the phone rang. I picked it up and heard Ron's voice. "Why have you stopped writing?" he asked. "I keep sending letters but I stopped receiving them from you." That's when we realized my mother was throwing his letters away!

To this day I'm ashamed to say that I never even got angry at her for doing such a terrible thing. I should have screamed and yelled, but I didn't. Where was my backbone? I should have run away. I should have refused to ever see her again! What was the matter with me? I failed Ron and myself.

I still argue with myself about it. After all, she was my mother, and she did have a hard life. And I was probably the only person who knew how badly she had suffered. Could I blame her for wanting me to be her princess, the daughter who would fulfill her dreams? How could I deny her that? So I wore the dresses she made for me and studied hard in school. I even planned to be the teacher she wanted me to be. I was her good girl. Nevertheless, when I learned she was throwing away Ron's letters, I got my own post office box.

My mother must have known we were writing again, because she took one more deadly action. Without telling me, she wrote a letter to Ron, explicitly asking him to stop writing or calling me. She said she didn't approve of our relationship and that I had to go to college and become a teacher before I would settle down. I didn't learn about that letter until many years later. All I knew was that Ron disappeared from my life.

We saw each other only one more time—as married people with young kids.

That brings us back to the morning in my kitchen when I spotted the letter from Ron. I can't tell you exactly why, but somehow I knew it was an important moment, perhaps because I had a decision to make. He had invited me to our high school reunion, and I had to say yes or no.

I knew that I *should* say no. All the signs pointed to that conclusion. I wanted to have sex with him, and that's adultery! No married woman should have thoughts like I had. Fred and I had a long history together, and even though he was hard to live with, I was committed to him. Besides, I knew my mother would turn over in her grave if I went. Anyway, I was too old for such an escapade. What would my children say?

I called Barbara, a friend from my college days who had become a therapist, and asked her to help me. We agreed to speak as friends. She knew I was a very good gardener, and she needed some help planning a perennial bed. So we began to speak regularly over the phone, though the truth be told, I was the one who did most of the speaking. I talked about how I yearned to recapture those early years. "Why should I deprive myself of Ron?" I asked repeatedly. "Certainly not out of loyalty to a husband who doesn't know the first thing about being intimate. Nor should I repeat the mistakes of the past. I let us be torn apart once and I don't want to do it again! And the children will understand. I've taught them better than to make simple judgments about anyone, let alone me."

Barbara repeatedly said that she could listen, but ultimately I had to find the answer to my dilemma inside myself, that no one could tell me what to do. And we talked about prayer as a route to gaining insight. So I prayed hard, listening for the right direction. And then I heard the words. *Love is the way.* Those words filled me up. My answer had come.

And then I bought my airline tickets. It's probably not surprising to you, but my depression lifted. I cleaned up the house and began to lose weight. It seemed I had found my courage once again.

I even tried to be honest with Fred. When he once again accused me of that "sidestep shuffle," I told him he was calling me a lazy good-for-nothing slave, and that it infuriated me. His reaction was quick and devastating. He recalled how I had often called him "an inhibited, boring, white lover." Those words made him feel as if all he would ever be for me was some distasteful notion of the white male. We were both hurting each other. The conversation made us feel a little closer.

The weekend of the reunion finally came, and I caught my first glimpse of Ron as I got off the airplane in Savannah. Yes, his hair was gray and his face showed years of wear, but he was still radiant. I felt the same strength in him I knew in our early years. Only it was deeper now, and more grounded.

"You look more beautiful than ever," he said. "I've imagined you over and over again, but none of those images come near the woman I see." Squeezing my hand, he added, "I can't tell you how happy I am that you're with me again."

We talked eagerly as we drove out to the home of a childhood friend who was hosting us for the weekend. Ron told me about his marriage, and the emptiness he felt after the children left. Still, he admitted that his was a good life, and he had lots of freedom to do his work. And I talked about Fred, saying much the same thing. But I didn't talk for long. This weekend was our chance to feel free of the present. If we let ourselves, we could come to each other as we were years ago, two very good friends.

The homecoming was like a fantasy come true. Vaguely familiar people, looking strange in their gray hair, emerged and disappeared in the school gym as if we were all in a mist. Only Ron and the music seemed real. We danced as if we had never parted. I knew then we would be lovers. It wouldn't be immediate; we had some thinking to do. But we both wanted it.

Fall had already arrived when I went down to Georgia the second time. This was for a beach weekend with the old high school group—or so I told Fred. In fact, it was the romantic getaway Ron and I had planned.

An old friend helped out by offering a secluded cabin in the dunes.

As soon as I saw Ron at the airport, I felt the excitement. It was almost too much to bear. I even had the impulse to turn and run back to the plane, but instead, I chuckled at my discomfort and paid close attention to the way his hand brushed the line of my cheek, moved down to touch my elbow, and finally took on the burden of my heavy bag. How jealous I was of that bag.

We bubbled with talk. "I'm in the midst of an effort to lobby the legislature for more money for the schools in our city," I began, "and my daughter is pregnant and due in May. I've promised to spend a few weeks with her after the baby comes. I love to take care of newborns."

"I bet you're a wonderful grandmother. How lucky this baby will be to have you," he reflected.

"I've just gotten a grant to do some research on hypertension," he added, catching me up. "But I'll take some time off next month so that my wife and I can go to San Francisco and see our daughter and her two kids. Tamara, the oldest, is giving a ballet recital we want to see."

"Look at us talking about our grandchildren," I laughed. "Is this what lovers of our age do?" We laughed with the joy of it. There seemed to be no end to what we had to share. And always, there was the glance that held the excitement and the touch that promised more. My body ached to feel his skin—the whole long length of his skin.

"Having held your breasts so many times in my dreams," he sighed, "I think I know exactly how they feel. But I can't wait any longer to feel them in real life."

I blushed as though I were a young girl and no one had ever talked to me like this. But then, I realized, no one ever had! Fred wouldn't even talk about sex, let alone touch me as suggestively as Ron did.

"Do you know what I dream about?" I asked. "Your hands. I love your hands. I imagine them on my breasts, on my stomach, gently stroking me. I ache for them."

We reached the house in the dark, searched for the key under the potted plant, and entered the cabin. There was no time to take the bags out of the car, to shop for food, or even to see if the water was running. There was no time for anything but us.

I ran my fingers down his spine and asked, "Do you like it when I do this?" His skin itself responded with a yes. When his lips approached me, seeming to ask if this was as exciting for me as it was for him, my whole body responded with the same yes.

We enveloped each other in bed, laughing at our good fit. And when I turned to lie on top of him, he smiled his delight. With trust and gentleness, we made the stranger within each of us friends, the frightened child within each of us safe. His reaching arms stroked in smooth and powerful caresses, my body arching in response. I felt alive again. And so the dark depths that might have engulfed us instead supported us. The lust that might have obliterated us instead sustained us. We rested in the danger, held by love as surely as currents of air hold the sea bird. And soon there was no turning back. Letting go of inhibition, I responded to each wave of excitement as it flowed up my spine, through my groin, and down to my toes.

A few hours later we awoke gleefully, like children amazed by their good fortune. But our lovemaking didn't stop. It continued in the long early morning walk on the miles of golden sand, in my attention to Ron's smile, and in his readiness to enjoy my laughter. We loved each other as the youngsters we used to be, and as the elders we were now.

Sometimes I would have a failure of courage and mock myself. "Do you see the wrinkles on my face? Do my large hips bother you?"

And he would say, "As for your hips, I love their fullness. They make our love-play feel especially luscious. Your wrinkles are another matter. They are the more of you that's been added over the years, so they make you even more special."

The weekend went by all too fast. On Sunday afternoon, lying in bed after making love, no longer able to keep the outside world at bay, it came back forcefully. "Let's not leave," I murmured as we clung to each other. "I love you so much. I can't bear the thought of separation."

Ron didn't respond right away, and I became anxious. "Where are you?" I asked. "What has happened? Don't you love me?"

"Yes, I do," he said with a certain flatness, the warmth I knew so well fading.

I needed some kind of reassurance, some confidence in our future.

"Tell me again. Tell me we'll find a way to be together. Tell me you'll always love me."

Ron's silence seemed impenetrable, his hands still and strange.

"Say it, Ron, please say you'll always love me."

"Try to think only of the moment," he finally answered. "That's best for now. Shouldn't we get up? It's almost time to leave for the airport."

"Yes," I said, more subdued now.

Still, I lingered a moment longer, watching him button his shirt and pull on his pants. Inside, I felt terribly devastated—and angry. How could he withdraw from me like that? Was I wrong to have been so open with him?

These thoughts led me to get up quickly and get dressed. Only then did I feel safe enough to speak. And my voice, when it finally came out, sounded more businesslike. "Ron, look at me. We need to talk about what just happened. I can't let this go by."

"What's the matter?" he asked, looking a little confused.

It was the fear I caught in his eyes that softened my anger. How could I be angry at such a dear soul? I could see that he didn't even know he had hurt me. But still, I had to tell him what I felt.

"You weren't very kind to me a moment ago when I asked you to tell me you would always love me. In fact, I would say you were mean."

"I'm so sorry," he quickly responded. "I'm so confused by all the feelings I'm having, I don't know what to say to you. I do love you. Of course I do. And I can't bear for you to leave now. The pain is terrible. And on top of that, I feel terrible putting you in a place like this."

Standing before me with tears in his eyes, he groaned, "I don't know what to do, Harriet, I don't know."

That's when I brushed my hand over his lips and whispered softly, "Shh. We don't have to figure it all out now. We'll find a way. I know we will." I smiled my love and ran my hands firmly over his shoulders, down his arms, and across his chest, tucking in his shirt, making sure he was still real.

Going home in the plane, the world still seemed like a dream; the intensity of the blue sky shocked me, and the sun cast a carpet of jewels on the ground below. Was this the way the world actually looked?

The next few months were hard. Should I leave my marriage and my home? Would that be best for Ron? What about our kids? The answers came over the next months as Ron and I conjured up many different ways to be together, wrote desperate letters, called each other with great urgency, and cried a lot—but managed to keep our affair secret. In this secrecy was the answer I had been waiting for.

Both of us had full lives. There were jobs and children and friends. And we knew that people would be hurt if we left. I had my new grand-child, and there was all that community work to be done. Ron had his patients to think about. We knew we would feel rootless without those old and very important connections. Our relationship, passionate as it was, was not an entire life.

In the end, and with great sadness, we decided not to uproot our-selves. Still, our love continued to add a subtle glow to life. Even though his marriage wasn't all he wished it was, somehow Ron managed. Know-ing I was a very special woman, I held myself with more self-respect. The course felt right, and was proven so, in the regard with which we held ourselves and the accomplishments that were to come.

Over the past decade we have written long, intimate letters about our personal doubts, our dreams, and our commitment to the friendship between us. And once every year I go back to Georgia to meet the "old group from high school" for another long summer weekend at the beach.

Birds make great sky-circles
of their freedom.
How do they learn it?

They fall, and falling,
they're given wings.

—RUMI

STITCHING THE WORLD TOGETHER WITH LOVE

Stories of *romantic love* enchant us. They lull us into the dream of a perfect union. As the story goes, two solitary souls search the wide earth for their true mates until the magic moment occurs, and then they live happily ever after. We're often so intrigued by these stories that we forget they're based on a myth. That's not to say that romantic love doesn't exist. It does, but only as the spark that brings people together, and not as an inevitable foundation for a long-term relationship.

There are at least two other equally important kinds of love: *spiritual love* and *loving kindness*. To my way of thinking, spiritual love is the force that knits together the larger whole in such a way that everything manifests within it in its own particular way. And what the Buddhists call loving kindness is borne of the insight that everything and everyone is of equal value in the larger, spiritual whole. Distinctions between good and bad, better and worse, are irrelevant.

In order to delve more deeply into the mystery of love, let's imagine a dance between the *I* that is each self and the *we* that is their union. From the perspective of each *I*, the dancers need to move as individuals in order to manifest themselves. From the perspective of the *we*, the dancers need to move together in order to create the couple. We call the *I-we* a polarity because it seems impossible to move separately and be together at the same time. Actually, it is possible. Indeed, each of the three kinds of love are choreographed so that this can happen. Let's look at how they do it.

Romantic love is a dream come true because the dance between the *I* and the *we* happens so easily at the beginning of a relationship. Lovers are often awed by how well they fit together. Their moods seem to match each other, their thoughts seem to resonate, even their tastes seem similar. At the same time, they're intrigued by the other's individuality. Lovers thrive, and they often assume their romance will last forever.

But it doesn't. As a relationship matures, lovers become aware that what's good for the *we* isn't always good for the *I*. So they worry that the obligations that come with a relationship will obliterate their individual selves. Alternatively, what's good for the *I* isn't always good for the *we*.

This makes lovers worry that their personal interests will obliterate the deep connection that the relationship offers, at least as a potential, and they'll be lonely again. This is the polarity that pits the *I* against the *we* and the *we* against the *I*.

It's all too easy for partners to be thrown into the clamor of hurt and anger when either the *I* or the *we* is neglected. If they deny each other the freedom to pursue their individuality, their relationship can feel like a prison. On the other hand, if their *we* is neglected, partners drift apart and possibly separate.

There are couples, the happy ones, who actually solve the *I-we* polarity. They do so because they don't resist either the *I* or the *we*; indeed, they move along a range of different degrees of closeness—from one side of the polarity to the other. This is possible only if they don't fear either the loss of self or the loss of the other. Deep down, it's fear that makes relationships so hard. Yet many couples find their way through that fear and so create a long-term romantic relationship.

Harriet and Ron are one example. Their tale is about a *we* that was found and lost several times in their youth but, fortunately, was given another chance. The love they found overcame geographical distance, a wrathful mother, existing marriages, and a bevy of children. But that wasn't the end of their trouble: having found each other, they had to face the opposite side of the *I-we* polarity. If they decided to live together, at least one of them would have to give up a rich individual life.

Fortunately for us all, Harriet and Ron's post–World War II generation invented a new American love story, one that loosened the couple from family or custom and was therefore more egalitarian than past love stories. This meant the *we* as well as the *I* was valuable. What a remarkable cultural achievement! It meant that Harriet could hold her desire for a union with Ron in one hand and her search for individual wholeness in the other, and then make choices—a freedom unknown in other times and other cultures. Sometimes she opted for *I*, sometimes for *we*. Love didn't capture Ron and Harriet; instead, they made an interesting choice.

By the time the story ended, they had decided to make room for their *we*, but only once a year. Was that enough? Perhaps, given their stage of life. The union they created kept them connected, with enough room to manifest the individual identities each had shaped over half a century. In this way, they transcended the *I-we* polarity that is at the heart of love.

I was honored to be asked to play a part in their lives. My part was essentially to be a witness, to listen to my dear friend's story as it occurred. Given my background as a therapist, I also helped her stay focused on the *I-we* polarity she and Ron had to solve. And I was delighted when they solved it so that the love she gave to Ron was also a love she gave to herself. It even seeped into the relationship with her grandchildren, her husband, and the many people she worked with in her community.

I recall visiting with Harriet once when she was filled with despair. I asked her to find that feeling in her body. She said her throat felt tight, and her eyes were almost tearing. Soon she was sobbing. The very best I could do for her at that moment was to help her direct some loving toward herself. And so I asked her to close her eyes, imagine one of her grandchildren, and find the feeling of warmth in her body that she felt for that child. Slowly, over the next half hour, she directed that feeling toward herself, and by the time she left her eyes were brighter and her back a little straighter. Most of us need to foster the capacity for greater self-love. It serves us in good stead as we try to live in relationships.

Now let's take a look at spiritual love. Great figures such as Christ, Moses, and the Buddha each spoke of a love that is built into the universe. Indeed, according to Christianity, God *is* love. According to Judaism, love is one with the act of creation. And compassion is at the heart of Buddhism. In all these spiritual traditions, love just is; there's nothing we have to do, or study, or earn, to find it. We simply need to be open to its existence.

Spiritual love also has the *I-we* polarity built into it. However, this is a love that transcends the polarity by holding the *I* and the *we* together. We're held in such a way that each planet, each goose, and each person has an individual identity within the larger spiritual whole. Not only that—we don't have to do anything, or be anyone special, to belong. There's no struggle.

Spiritual love doesn't discriminate; everything and everyone is of equal value. Everything and everyone is loved. That's because we inter-are. According to this insight, the rose in my garden and I are entirely different beings, and yet we are also one. The rose contains the energy of the sun, minerals from the earth, and water from rain. It develops according to codes inscribed in the DNA that is held in common by all beings. I, too, contain the energy of the sun, minerals from the earth, and water from rain. I also am the product of that DNA. All life is made up of the same nonliving elements. All life follows the same basic rules. Look deeply enough into the rose and you will feel the connection. Every one of us takes a separate form, and yet we live in and through each other. We inter-are.

Here's an example: One day while standing at the corner of Broadway and Forty-second Street in New York City, I became aware that though there were crowds of people maneuvering to cross, they only rarely collided with one another. If you watched, you would see how people make way for the old man who walks slowly, the child who darts quickly, or the bicyclist going at double the speed of anyone else. Without being aware of it, the people of New York City create brief but mutually beneficial relationships; they care enough not to bump into each other. It's all very complicated, but even a poodle can do it. Each person in a crowd, like each fish in a school, is both separate and connected within the larger whole. Spiritual love just is. This is how it solves the *I-we* dilemma.

And now we come to a third kind of love. Buddhists call it loving kindness. In an effort to live in an awareness of inter-being, compassion arises. We know that if the green plants on this earth start to fail, we, too, will fail. If the human race on this earth starts to fail, each of us will also fail. To nurture and protect ourselves, we need to nurture and protect other beings. Our well-being is dependent on their well-being. Indeed, we have to care for the larger whole itself. Our well-being is dependent on its well-being. Once we let go of the focus on the self, it's but another small step to feel loving kindness for the beached whale or the poor child who has nothing to eat. It feels remarkably good.

There are many of us on this earth who practice loving kindness, whether it takes the form of protecting the environment, serving food to the hungry, or caring for the criminal. Unlike romantic love, loving kindness doesn't expect anything in return. It is a more inclusive love; you needn't have a certain kind of body, a particular amount of money in the bank, or any special status to be loved. Nor does this love have to be anything more than a momentary experience. You can see a rose, look into a friend's eyes, or hold a newborn and simply, freely, feel the warmth of loving kindness spread through the body. It just is.

How does loving kindness solve the dilemma that exists between the *I* and the *we*? Through insight and skillful behavior. Having had the insight that love is built into the larger spiritual whole, we cultivate the human capacity to live within that love, offering it freely and without any need to own the other. In this way, loving kindness offers union without denying the needs of individuals. Harriet and I often shared a loving kindness meditation when we talked on the telephone. It helped her love herself as well as Ron—and understand that their union had to nurture both the *I* and the *we*. That was a way out of the polarity.

Loving kindness also comes with the insight that there's enough love to go around, so we don't have to hoard it. A modern fairy tale that I heard many years ago actually describes this loving kindness. Here's how it goes:

Once upon a time long, long ago, there was a land where everyone felt loved. That was because people hugged each other freely and without expecting anything in return. So no one, absolutely no one, felt deprived. Children knew without being told that the more hugs they gave, the more they would get back. Nobody took advantage of another; people were compassionate when others were hurt and generous with their wealth. All was well in the world.

One day a cruel witch came into town and cast an evil spell. It took the form of plastic fuzzies that she sold, claiming they were much better to give than warm hugs. So persuasive was she that people bought a lot of them from her. At first, the plastic fuzzies were fun to have around and give because they were multicolored and shimmered in the sun. However, they cost a lot of money, which meant some people had a lot while others had only a few. And because people were afraid of running out of their plastic fuzzies, they began to give them away only sparingly. Eventually, everyone began to get sick, children hated school, and the economy sputtered. There seemed to be no reason to smile anymore.

Then a good witch came into town. She began to whisper into people's ears, "Hugs never run out. You can give away as many of your hugs as you like, and you'll always have enough. Besides, they're good for you and everyone else!"

At first, only the children heard this good news, but when they began to smile and laugh again, the adults caught on. Soon the economy was thriving, everyone's health improved, and all the children did well at school. The cruel witch's spell had been lifted. And people felt thankful.

At one time or another, most of us have felt love freely given; perhaps it was in the form of help from a teacher, the trust of a friend, or the caring of a parent. This is loving kindness. It's a radical acceptance of inter-being. We are all connected. To respond with gratitude to loving kindness is to enlarge our capacity for love.[1]

You can cultivate loving kindness just like you cultivate awareness. That's what the next meditation offers. Here's what happens:

The first instruction is to think of someone you love or to try to see that person on the screen in front of your closed eyes. Either will do. Then I'll ask you to search in your body for the feeling of love, caring, or warmth that you feel toward that person. If you can't find it, simply imagine it.

Then I'll ask you to repeat three phrases as a chant: *May he or she be free from danger. May he or she know physical and mental well-being. May he or she know happiness.* Please decide for yourself whether these words work for you or whether you need to choose others. And substitute a name for *he* or *she*. Whatever words you choose, try to say them with awareness and intention. When you do so, they will be a force all their own. You will then use the entire sequence as you send your loving kindness to other people.

There's much to learn from a meditation on loving kindness. And, if you immerse yourself fully, it can feel remarkably fulfilling because you're touching love inside yourself.

He who binds himself to a joy
Does the winged life destroy.

But he who kisses the joy as it flies
Lives in eternity's sunrise.

—WILLIAM BLAKE

A Meditation on Loving Kindness

Settle into a comfortable place, perhaps a favorite lounge chair. Since this is a meditation on pleasure, it's important not to let minor difficulties get in the way.

When you're ready, **imagine** *a person you love . . . a dear friend . . . a parent . . . a spouse . . . a baby. Perhaps you will* **see** *a fuzzy image of that person. Maybe not. That's fine . . . either imagining or seeing will do.*

Now scan your body and try to detect the feeling of loving kindness. Perhaps it's a warm glow inside your chest . . . maybe it's a stillness or a sense of well-being.

Then silently say to yourself:

May [name] be free from danger.

May [name] know physical and mental well-being.

May [name] know happiness.

Hold this person in your awareness for five minutes, while repeating the chant.

When you're ready, once again **imagine** *or* **see** *the person you love, and feel the warmth that's associated with him or her. Then* **imagine** *or* **see** *someone else . . . someone who needs your loving kindness. Perhaps your loving kindness will emerge as caring . . . or a feeling of warmth or tenderness in the*

*body. Alternatively, you may imagine that caring or warmth. Then direct it
toward that person who needs your loving kindness. And **hear** yourself say:*

> *May [name] be free from danger.*
>
> *May [name] know physical and mental well-being.*
>
> *May [name] know happiness.*

For five minutes, hold this person in your awareness and repeat the chant.

❀

*Again, **imagine** or **see** the person you love, and **imagine** or **feel** the warmth
of loving kindness he or she arouses inside you. Direct that loving kindness
to someone who has hurt you . . . or offended you. Perhaps this warmth will
take the form of a greater acceptance of the person . . . even some caring . . .
perhaps not. Nevertheless, **hear** yourself say:*

> *May [name] be free from danger.*
>
> *May [name] know physical and mental well-being.*
>
> *May [name] know happiness.*

Let this person be in your awareness for five minutes, and recite the chant.

❀

*Now **imagine** or **see** the person you love. And **imagine** or **feel** the warmth of
loving kindness in your body . . . perhaps some caring . . . or compassion . . .
Then direct that feeling toward yourself. If you can't find the warmth . . .
that's okay. Instead, you might imagine yourself being held in your own arms.
And **hear** yourself say:*

> *May I be free from danger.*
>
> *May I know physical and mental well-being.*
>
> *May I know happiness.*

*Perhaps you will feel uncomfortable with the meditation. Maybe you
think it doesn't make sense. All that is important, but for now, simply set
those responses aside. See or imagine yourself . . . and feel or imagine the
warmth or tenderness of loving kindness flowing toward yourself.*

*You, too, need loving kindness. And the miracle is . . . you can give it to
yourself.*

For five minutes, direct this loving kindness toward yourself.

❀

In one last effort, on the screen in front of your eyes, begin by **imagining** *or* **seeing** *the person you love. Feel or imagine the warmth for him or her. Then* **imagine** *or* **see** *the whole earth . . . and saturate the whole earth with that warmth. Finally,* **hear** *yourself say:*

> *May the whole earth be free from danger.*
>
> *May all beings on this earth know physical and mental well-being.*
>
> *May all beings on this earth know peace.*

Send the whole earth those good wishes . . . let them spread like the rays of the sun until they reach every sentient being.

Send your warmth . . . your compassion . . . your loving kindness out into the world.

Enjoy the expansiveness of the endeavor. Relax into the pleasure of sending loving kindness to the whole earth.

❀

When you're ready, slowly open your eyes. And sit quietly in the warm glow of loving kindness.

Try this meditation when you're feeling disconnected from others, unloved, unloving of yourself, or trapped in a troublesome emotion, or when you are aware of the great suffering in the world. As you learn how to access love inside you, it will be easier to find love when you need it.

May all beings know loving kindness.

Training for Awareness

1. Imagine or see someone you love. Direct loving kindness toward that person. Repeat the chant.

2. Imagine or see someone who needs your love. Direct loving kindness toward that person. Repeat the chant.

3. Imagine or see someone who has hurt you. Direct loving kindness toward that person. Repeat the chant.

4. Imagine or see yourself. Direct loving kindness toward yourself. Repeat the chant.

5. Imagine or see the whole earth. Direct loving kindness toward the earth. Repeat the chant.

Nine

Marcia Wants to Live
until She Dies

I am dying. Probably not today or tomorrow, but the hard truth is I am dying. My oncologist told me I might even live for six more months; but doctors stretch the time when speaking to patients about death, so I probably have a month or two less. The test results after the second round of chemotherapy just came back. The treatment didn't stop the cancer's progress.

My husband, Ben, held my hand tightly as we heard the news. I don't think either of us took a full breath until we found our way out of that office and into our car. And then we cried.

"We have to get another opinion," he said. "There must be something else we can do."

"No, Ben," I said, with a sad strength that surprised me. "I don't want to. Medicine doesn't have the answer. We both know that. Besides, I don't want any more poison dripping into my veins or aseptic hospital rooms, and please, God, no procedures of last resort. I want to be home with you and Dorothy. I want to live until I die. Please, let's just go home."

"All right, honey. Let's go home to our baby," he said sadly. "We'll talk about it later."

We drove in silence, our minds going their separate ways, our hands tightly interwoven. My tears could have filled a riverbed. It was unfathomable to me that I was leaving my two-year-old daughter. How could it be? It didn't make sense. Just the idea was more than I could bear, which is probably why it kept slipping away, only to return a moment later with another stab of pain. All this upset must have put me in a state of shock, because the next thing I knew the scene outside the car window turned very still, silent, and exceptionally clear. The hum of the car's motor filled my ears, and the blue of the sky astounded me. Against that background, a hawk circled slowly, silently, gliding ever upward on a current of air. For a brief moment, I was that lone bird, held by the great wind, immersed in the wondrous beauty of it all. From somewhere deep inside my body came an overwhelming yearning to hold my baby, which drew me back to the earth. Strange to say, I felt not just sadness on the return but also some kind of aching joy. The moment passed quickly, and I was left wondering why the image appeared. What did it have to do with my dying?

That's when I swore to live my dying as fully as possible, squeezing the very last drop of juice out of life. I would live until I died, and maybe dying would become a spiritual path. But what did that mean?

Glancing toward Ben as he made a smooth turn onto the highway that would take us home, I became aware of his tall, athletic frame and the perfection of his clearcut profile. What would this do to him? He was such a capable man, so able to make things happen. But could he manage losing me? Would he fall apart? Or would he find someone else? It wouldn't be long before another woman would catch sight of the easy informality of him, the shock of black hair that wouldn't quite stay in place, the shy glance when he was caught unaware. When an image of Ben and another woman embracing came into my mind, I let out a cry.

"What's the matter?" Ben asked.

"I can't talk about it," I answered, adding still another tear-saturated tissue to the pile on my lap.

"Don't keep me out, Marcia," he pleaded. "It's hard enough to be going through this without you putting a wall between us."

He was right, I thought. I should tell him, but all I could do was cry hysterically. So he pulled over to the side of the road and held me. To my astonishment, he had sensed that I was thinking about him and another woman.

"Don't worry," he said. "It's you I love, sick or well. I'll always be with you—even after you die. But I hope that's not going to happen for a long time." And so we cried together.

"Ben," I said, finally finding my voice, "remember when we first learned that I had breast cancer, and how we promised each other that we wouldn't ever become victims of it?"

"Yes," he recalled, "or victims of the medical profession."

"I would like us to do the same with my death. I want to live it as fully as I lived the illness. There's no point in succumbing now. Dying can be a spiritual path, Ben. We can both learn from it. Let's live it fully."

"I'm afraid you're saying that you're ready to give up on staying alive," Ben responded, once again in tears. "Please don't do that, Marcia, please. Dorothy and I need you. We don't want you to leave us. I can't stand even the thought of it."

"Oh, Ben," I cried, "I don't want to. In the worst way I don't want to. But I've got to face what's happening to me. Being a writer, I'm used to digging into life. I can't give that up now and let myself become a blubbering casualty. I want to know what dying is about."

We were both quiet for a while, and then this man I loved added quietly: "Marcia, this is *your* life. I'll be with you in whatever way feels right to you. We've done the illness well. I'm proud of that. And we'll do whatever comes next just as well."

"I have a suggestion," he said, his dark brown eyes brightening. "You've always said that writing is a way of thinking for you. And you're good at it. Why not use that skill to watch what's happening? It might help all three of us."

I knew immediately he was right. Writing was just the tool I needed. For as long as I was able, I would catch glimpses of this spiritual path for myself and my family. And if I couldn't hold a pencil, I would use a tape recorder. Maybe others would find it helpful.

Actually, what you are reading now is the result of my words and Ben's editing. I truly hope you can stay with my one last effort—and learn what I learned along the way.

Soon we were home, and Dorothy was in my arms. Touching her sweet soft skin, it came to me that I didn't have to *find* that spiritual path. Living my life fully in the awareness of death *was* the path. It led us to live in the moment.

In a sense, even Dorothy's home birth had taken place on the path. We weren't then quite so aware of death as we were now, but we were in the moment. Ben and I did it together. With a midwife presiding, there weren't any white gowns, blank walls, face masks, or mind-numbing drugs to suppress this most sacred of acts. It was just Ben and me, and the midwife. I wish you could have seen the way we all worked together to open the way for Dorothy.

Ben was best of all. Sitting on the bed right next to my head, he sensed the contractions rise, peak, and subside and breathed through them with me. When they got serious, he held my shoulders and we rode those contractions for all they were worth. He even found ways to make me laugh when I needed some humor to manage the pain. We cried together when we saw the first patch of baby hair reflected in a well-placed mirror, and what a sense of glory when, after a few momentous pushes, Dorothy's head, her chin, and then her shoulders emerged. Truly, Ben and I gave birth to Dorothy.

Fortunately, we were able to take off six whole weeks in maternity/paternity leave to tend to her. At first it was as if all three of us were inside some big womb. Ben and I spent long hours lying in bed, the baby between us, our sleep schedule merging with hers so that the difference between day and night was almost lost. It was dreamlike to be immersed in all those bodily fluids—sweet breast milk intermingling with the sweat of our bodies. Ben called it baby bliss. In the blink of an eye, however, that entire experience was gone. The tiny little infant was just a memory.

In another blink of the eye, Dorothy was one year old, sitting in her high chair in the midst of grandparents and friends. I remember seeing everyone's eyes trained on her as she gleefully tried to blow out the candles. With a little help from me, she did it. As she looked up, I caught the sense of triumph in her eyes.

A year later, on a table right next to me, sat a picture of that birthday scene. Ben looked particularly appealing in his black sweater and jeans. I was the image of health, tall, lean, with long, thick red hair hanging loose down my back and a happy smile on my face. Ever mindful that my large breasts not attract too much attention, I was wearing one of my loose tops. Not only one year had gone; so had that attractive young woman.

The day after that party, I discovered a very small lump in the lower left quadrant of my right breast. There had been other lumps in the past, so I didn't feel like a foolish optimist concluding it probably was a cyst. Besides, I took care of myself. I was a vegetarian and had a daily exercise routine. Ben often joked, "Marcia is our in-house nutrition consultant."

Nevertheless, I called my gynecologist, got the necessary tests, and went in to have a biopsy. A few days later I was back sitting in her office expecting to hear that it was nothing. Instead, she told me this time it was for real. It wasn't just a cyst. I had cancer of a rare and rapidly growing type, and it had already spread to my lymph nodes. How ironic, with all my healthy living, and my conscious avoidance of caffeine, sweets, and saturated fats, that I should be the one to have breast cancer. I could have eaten tons of junk food for all it mattered!

The only other memory I have of those early days, before I started my journal, was sitting in bed late one night, with my tears and my worries tumbling out: "I'm scared, Ben. This might be terrible. It might even mean my death."

"I know you're worried. I am, too," Ben offered. "But there's good medical care out there these days. We'll find a way to get you well, Marcia. We have to."

"I'm afraid I'll need you too much. I don't want you to feel trapped by an invalid. Besides, life is so hectic as it is. How are we ever going to manage my cancer, your job, and Dorothy?"

We held each other close as Ben reassured me, even answering questions I hadn't been able to ask. "I love you more than words can say. I don't want you to ever doubt that. I'm here for you. We'll both keep our attention on getting you well. And I want to be part of the decision-making process. Don't leave me out. Just tell me if I'm too bossy."

We laughed, knowing that each of us could be that way. "I really want you to be with me," I said. "I'll feel safer that way. Who knows, maybe we'll sail through this."

Later that night he added: "Just you wait and see, we'll find a way to defeat this thing. We're capable of getting you the best that medicine has to offer. Anyway, the love we feel for each other and for Dorothy is the most powerful treatment of all."

God, I love that man! How did I ever get so lucky as to find him?

I don't need to tell yet another cancer treatment story; by this time you know about chemotherapy and its side effects. But I do want to describe how Ben and I worked together, because I'm proud of it. Our first decision was to give ourselves the reward of a fabulous vacation in Italy after the treatment was over. Tuscany was our place of choice. Ben brought home some travel books and even began cooking in the style of the region.

We also learned about cancer together. My oncologist, Dr. Anita Greenfield, clued me in on Web sites I could use to do research, and I made use of my medical friends to network with people who had the information we needed. No way would we let the medical establishment deprive us of decision making.

But that was not all. I couldn't shake the fear that my body wouldn't be able to manage the chemo, and that Ben wouldn't be able to put up with me. So I found a therapist. She helped me understand that these discouraging thoughts were simply my worries, and that I also had positive, even brave thoughts as well. And they were just as important. For instance, most of the time I really did think I had the strength to get through the treatment and that the cancer would let go of me. I began to call those thoughts my convictions. Then I learned how to practice replacing my worries with my convictions. It helped.

There were also some decisions to make, such as deciding whom I wanted to tell that I had cancer. Not an easy problem. My first impulse was to hide it from all the doom and gloom people I knew, but ultimately I decided to do the opposite—tell everybody. That would offer me more of the support I needed. It was a good strategy for everyone except my mother.

She was the hardest of all to tell. My father had died of lung cancer about six years before, and I knew she would be very upset if she knew about me. So I decided not to tell her. But then she called sounding worried. She had spoken to Ben, who wasn't his usual upbeat self, and she sensed something was wrong. Maybe because I was tired or perhaps because I ached for a mother's care, I couldn't stop myself from telling her what was happening. It was actually a relief. I could feel my body relax. And I was happy when she said she wanted to help.

Ben and I decided to ask her to stay with us during the chemotherapy to help out, and she quickly agreed. Imprinted in my mind is the picture of her cooking and cleaning in my kitchen, her chunky body covered by an old housecoat, her frizzy, grey hair usually undone. I couldn't ask for a more devoted helper. She was especially loving of Dorothy, who grew quite close to her. However, I remember lying in bed one day, nauseous, miserable, hearing the two of them chatter in the next room, and feeling jealous. I wanted to be the one talking to Dorothy. She was replacing me in my daughter's heart.

That's not the only thing that bothered me. My mother was wearing a frown on her face, showing that she was worrying her way through the day. And she cried a lot. In the morning, her eyes were red and sleepless. That made me feel guilty. Would I ever find a way through this morass of feelings?

"Why are you crying, Mom?" I asked one morning.

"Because you're so sick," she answered. "Because you don't take care of yourself well enough. Because I made chicken soup for you last night and you refused to eat it. You're just like your father was, stubborn, and look where it got him! You have to start eating what I cook for you!"

"Mom, don't you get it? I'm a vegetarian. I don't eat chicken!"

"I know," she said, "that's the problem! How can you expect to get well on what you eat?"

After one of these so-called conversations I was at my wit's end. Talk about being irrational! No amount of explaining helped when it came to my mother. After that brief conversation, I explicitly asked her not to bring chicken or any other meat into the house—but she did it anyway. And she gave it to Dorothy!

However, I really didn't have the energy to fight her. Besides, Dorothy felt safe when she was around, and Ben needed the time at work. So I retreated to my bedroom. There was nothing else I could do.

Finally, wonder of wonders, the chemotherapy and the six weeks of radiation were actually over. I had another round of life, blessed life. It's impossible to fully tell you how much the morning light meant to me . . . the symphony of the crickets . . . the whoosh of the wind . . . Dorothy's giggle when we played peek-a-boo—all the small things that made my heart soar.

The three of us went out to dinner that night. Ben and I drank champagne. Dorothy had her apple juice.

Life went back to normal, not pre-cancer normal but something that might be called post-cancer extraordinary-normal. Sure there was work and play and all the worry about any small ache in my body. But we also took that trip to Italy.

Three glorious weeks! We rented what was once a small farmhouse not too far from Florence, and Dorothy marched her way through town after town, her gleeful face attracting more attention than we ever thought possible. Grown men stopped in the middle of the street to play with her; mothers asked if she could have a piece of candy. With Dorothy around, we didn't need to know how to speak Italian. Parents have a universal language.

My senses were wide open. I remember waking up to the cool fresh air coming through our bedroom window and the sounds of birds, chickens, and an occasional person tending the supports in the vineyard down in the valley below. Ben and I fell in love again during those early mornings before Dorothy got up. It was a new kind of love, a post-cancer extraordinary-love we would say to each other, as we learned our bodies all over again. Never before had we paid such close attention to the simple feeling of being hugged. I relished being encircled in his arms with my head tucked into his neck, our bodies touching down the whole length of me. He delighted in resting his head on my breast, with my arms holding him fully, tightly. When Dorothy woke up and came toddling into the room for a few precious moments, she settled in between us in still another kind of hug.

On the last morning of the vacation, when we were trying to get ourselves to the airport on time, I was particularly aware of death and the briefness of our lives. While Ben was packing the car, Dorothy and I looked around the house for lost objects, said good-bye to the cat, and locked the door. Then I made the mistake of simply picking her up and putting her into the car seat, as if she were another bag of clothes. Once she caught on, she objected with ever increasing intensity. "No, me do it!" she cried, "Me do it!" By the time she was strapped in, her wails could be heard across the valley. So with an internal groan, I lifted her out of the seat and put her down on her own two feet outside the car. And then I stood back, closed my eyes, breathed deeply, and waited until she slowly managed to climb up into the car seat all by herself.

"Me do it!" she announced proudly.

Watching my child smile back at me proudly from the depths of her car seat, I had another one of those exceptionally clear spiritual moments. I saw that Ben, Dorothy, and I, the lush vineyard below, and the cloudless sky above were part of a vast and very beautiful Cézanne painting. And I ached with the sweet sadness of it all, knowing that all too soon this exquisite scene would be nothing but another faded memory.

Afterward, I realized the vision was intense precisely because it stood out in relief against my lingering dread of cancer. My cancer was a doorway to those heightened experiences. I usually don't like it when people say their cancer helped them, but the truth is, I would never have had those moments without cancer.

Then came the day when Ben and I went to see my oncologist for the results of my one-year checkup. We hadn't seen Anita for six months and looked forward to saying hello, so we came in smiling, joking, fully expecting that this would be a day of triumph. But looking into her face, I knew right away the news was bad. The X rays showed that the cancer had returned.

Given the type of cancer, she said, the odds weren't good. The cells were reproducing too fast. And at the moment, there was no sure way to stop them. They were already invading my lungs.

Was this to be my fate? Sitting in that office, for the first time I seriously considered the possibility that I would die. But the thought was only momentary. I quickly dismissed it, fearing it would rob me of the will to live. And that will was something I had to maintain. Losing Ben would be terrible, but losing my baby girl would be more painful than words could ever say.

When I tuned back into the conversation, Anita was suggesting a still more powerful round of chemotherapy. It was one of those new medications, of great promise, but untested. She thought I was a good candidate because I was young and strong. It would all but destroy my white blood cells, but my health could be managed by keeping me in the aseptic environment of a hospital for as long as necessary. To get the treatment, I would have to go to a particular hospital in New York.

My first reaction was to refuse. I didn't want to spend whatever time I had left on this earth being sick. And I certainly didn't feel sure of my body's capacity to fight the cancer. I was tired even at the thought of it. Nor did I believe in medicine's capacity to help. But looking over at Ben, who was trying hard to say nothing and give me the room to make my own decision, I knew how much he wanted me to try to live. I owed it to him and Dorothy to keep on trying. At that moment I also realized that someday I might have to fight for the freedom to die—even with Ben.

But this was not the time for that. How could I say no to even the slimmest chance that this treatment would save my life? I had to devote all my energy to living. So I agreed to the next chemotherapy treatment.

Anita, Ben, and I began to figure out how to manage it. I knew I didn't want my mother to be a part of the plan this time. I didn't want my energy drained by the struggle with her. Ben squeezed my hand in affirmation when he heard my little speech. Anita knew someone who not only could help out with Dorothy but also had experience managing some of the side effects of this treatment. But I also said no to that offer. I didn't want a stranger in the house.

Somehow I believed that I would be able to manage. It was true, during the first few weeks of the treatment I could, with some help from Ben. But soon, too soon, I got very weak, and Ben really did have to go to work. So we hired Emily for the daytime shift. Frankly, it was a relief to have a stranger taking care of me. There was no one for me to protect. I could just be sick.

My mother still came to visit once a week. I couldn't deprive her of that. But the visit took its toll. Once she came quietly into my room when I was half asleep, peered down at me, and cried silently.

When I asked what was the matter, she spoke as if she were a young, frightened child. "I'm afraid you're going to die, Marcia."

What could I say? She had the knack of tuning in to my deepest fear and hurling it in my face. My impulse was to tell her to shut up, but how could I do that when she cared so much? Besides, it wouldn't stop her. I didn't have much control of anything, let alone of her. It was good to know I had done better with my own life. I was more capable of being intimate with my loved ones. And Dorothy, I hoped, would do even better. She might even be able to let a woman take care of her more easily.

Soon it became difficult to manage my mother's visits. I was irritable. Why did I have to take care of her, especially at a time like this? Would it ever be my turn? Lying in bed after one of her visits, I remembered how often I was sick as a child, how often I stayed home from school. Was it to take care of me or to take care of her? I wondered. Then I recalled being sixteen and really ill, with a bad stomachache. When my mother wanted me to stay home, I lied and said I was well enough to go to school. I insisted on taking care of myself. And so I did, from then on.

When Ben came home that night, we talked it over and decided to ask my mother to visit for no more than a half hour, once a week. When she came, I would tell Emily whether I felt well enough to see her. It felt right. I had to do it.

Late that night I woke up after a very clear dream. In it, I saw a bag sitting right next to me, on the floor beside the bed. The bag was white and made of something durable, maybe canvas. Somehow I knew my mother's bones were in that bag. Bone of my bone, they were the essence of her, the woman who gave birth to me, who held me, cleaned me, fed me. Those bones had nothing to do with her worry, her fear that I wasn't strong enough, or her inability to meet me. The bones were the best of my mother, her love for me. And that was a treasure. "Thank you, Mom," I whispered. "Thank you."

The fear of losing me was cycling not only through my mother's consciousness, but through Dorothy's as well. If I happened to be out of sight for a moment, she would scream as if I were never coming back. If she happened to wake up in the middle of the night, she would yell out in panic. "Mommy, Mommy, where are you?" No matter how badly I felt, I rushed to her side and held her tightly. I wondered how long I would be able to.

And when our fish, Platty, died, Ben quickly went out and bought another so that she wouldn't have to face the loss. I laugh at that now. In her own way, this child of ours already knew about attachment and loss. She'd been working on that problem from the day she was born! Dorothy would make it through life. She was strong enough.

As was expected, after a month or so my white blood count dropped low enough to raise the risk of infection, so it was time to move into the hospital. That meant leaving the comfort of my home so I could go to New York and submit to the medical establishment. After all the years spent trying to find an alternative approach to health, I would be housed, sick and weak, deep within the beast.

Ben and I tried to dispel the beast's power by making my room as homelike as possible. We put pictures of the family on the wall; the African violet plants that usually sat in our dining room were on the window ledge; and my computer was near the bed so I could send e-mail to friends—if I felt well enough. However, anyone who came to see me had to wear a mask. I still felt unreal, cut off, exiled.

I wasn't in the hospital long before they stopped the treatment and sent me home.

And so we come back to the moment in time when I began to write this story: that visit to Anita after my second round of chemo, when the test results came back and she told us the treatment hadn't worked.

There was no escaping it this time; I had no choice but to accept the reality that I was dying. At first I did remarkably well. Insight after insight guided me. Ben was close by, grounding me when I needed it, encouraging me to continue. That was when I took this dying of mine to be a spiritual path.

But after forty-eight hours, I crashed. "How could it be?" I cried out loud to Ben, shedding oceans of tears. "All that suffering to no avail. How could this happen to me? What did I do to deserve it? Dorothy is just two and a half, and it's not fair!" Then, bitterly, "No God I can think of would do this."

Ben tried to console me, offering the hope that all was not lost. "We'll find another way, we will."

The tears streaming down my face and onto the pillow, I moaned, "Don't fool yourself anymore, Ben. My body isn't able to resist the cancer. The truth is, I'm going to die. I need you to accept it . . . because that will make it easier for Dorothy and me to do the same."

"Marcia, we don't really know what will happen. There are stories of other people with cancers that stopped growing for no apparent reason. You have to keep up your hope. We need you."

"Please," I begged, "if I am to live this dying well, I can't deny the fact that it's happening. I *am* dying. If I should *stop* dying, I'll do something different."

"My mind says you're right," he answered, holding me close enough for his tears to blend with mine, "but my heart won't let me accept it. I know it's not right for me to try to tell you what to do or think. It's your life and your call. I'll do whatever you wish. But just try to keep a little corner of your mind free enough to believe in miracles."

"I will, my darling, I will. But please, please give me the freedom to die in my own way. Let me be me in this awful illness. And be strong for me."

But there were limits to Ben's strength. Even though he was trying to keep going, he began to collapse inside. More and more, he didn't quite make it into work. It seemed irrelevant to him. And I would wake up in the middle of the night to see him watching me, tears in his eyes. Worse still, he began to hover around me during the day, urging me to eat, asking if I was comfortable, trying unsuccessfully to make me laugh. He was a mess.

At first I felt sorry for him, and I tried to be loving and kind. But all this hovering made me irritable, almost claustrophobic. I was more worried about him than about myself. Just when I needed him to be strong, he wasn't.

"Ben," I begged each morning, "please go to work. I love you so much, but I can't bear the way you're hovering. You can't save me that way. I wish you could, but you can't. Please, you have to continue to be strong for the family. Please, Ben, be strong."

But each night he stayed awake to watch me. And each morning he broke into tears at the thought of leaving to go to work. "I just can't face the day without you. I can't leave. I can't."

That's when I called my therapist, Barbara, and asked for help. She came to the house that very night—and the three of us met in my bedroom. We cried, and we talked, and we cried again until we were exhausted. Then we meditated together. And we found our strength. Ben's backbone seemed to straighten as he acknowledged that he had to keep going, that Dorothy and I needed him. And I felt even more sure that I didn't have the strength to take care of him.

With Barbara's continued help, he managed to go to work on most days, but more important to me, he didn't hover quite as much.

And so I prepared for my death. Early in the morning, when I still had some energy, I would spend fifteen to twenty minutes making audiotapes for Dorothy. For one, I read some of her favorite bedtime stories, including *Good Night Moon* and *Curious George*. For another, for Dorothy when she was four or five, I read one of my favorite books, *The Wizard of Oz*.

By the time I got to making her a tape for her third birthday, however, breathing was more difficult, and I could record only for a few moments. But I had to do it. Even though it was a few months away, the celebration would probably come after my death. It was now or never. So I sang happy birthday to her and told her the story of her birth. I also explained that I would always be with her in spirit. If she wanted to hear my voice, she could always put on the tape. But she might even be able to hear the memory of my voice without the tape. I loved her and always would.

With Emily's help, I made a tape for Ben. It held some of my memories: the joy of meeting him, some of the good times we had together. With lots of tears, I also said that I wanted him to find someone else. Not that she would ever take my place, but I felt strongly that he and Dorothy needed someone who could love them both.

I became tired, so tired I didn't even want to talk. Instead, I was drawn toward the sound of Gustav Mahler's deeply emotional music. And sometimes, when I felt able, I liked to listen to Aaron Copland. His soaring energy was almost enough to lift me into the sky with him.

At night, after Dorothy went to sleep, Ben would read to me, just for a little while. The sound of his voice hummed inside my head. More and more, however, I preferred the quiet. The sound of everyday life that came through the window was my music. And something as simple as the shadow on the wall could fill me with such delight that I would chuckle.

"What are you thinking?" Ben often asked after a long period of silence.

When I felt a little stronger, I tried to tell him. "It's beautiful, Ben. And so peaceful, this world of ours, once you get away from the noise. I imagine it's what death will be. And that's not so bad."

After a moment of silence, he whispered hoarsely, "You were always the precocious one, Marcia. Remember the stories your mother tells of how you played Mozart on the piano when you were in second grade? And didn't your mother call you Einstein because you figured out how to count before you could speak in sentences? You have a history of learning remarkable things before your time." We laughed wryly, which was just what I needed. I looked into his eyes and told him how proud I was of him, how much I loved him. He broke into tears again, but somehow I was all right with them. I just held his hand.

I had to admit that every day I was feeling weaker. My cough had become vicious. It came in spasms that left me in a sweat and exhausted. And it was ever harder to breathe. I was so glad I had Emily to help me during the day. However, the nights were hardest of all. I felt awful putting Ben through my long coughing spells and the night sweats. Emily taught me to breathe into a paper bag when I felt panic to increase the amount of carbon dioxide I took in. Ben helped me do it at night. I used morphine to take the edge off the pain, but not too much. I didn't want to numb my mind.

Dorothy would come to visit me during the day, and I was happy to see her, but also relieved when Emily took her away. I was so preoccupied with my body that my daughter was fading from my consciousness. When it came to me that I wouldn't know what career she would choose, or the man she would marry, it was somehow okay. My human connections were slowly unraveling. I was entering into another world, and, surprisingly, it was comforting. Within it I could rest. Odd beings we are, thinking we should deny our very deaths rather than simply being part of the miracle.

In a dream I saw Ben calling to me, wanting me. I tried to explain that I was too tired to come. He heard me and smiled his acceptance as he faded away. "Oh, Ben, dear Ben, if only we could be together," I heard myself say.

There were more moments of peace, moments when my internal life became extraordinarily clear, pregnant with energy. In the middle of one painful night I was swept away by the wind . . . supported by the up-drafts much like the hawks that I loved to watch. The pain seemed far away, quite bearable. Even the tears stopped. Just the wind remained and I was one with it. I was letting go. And it wasn't really all that bad.

Hearing people talk at a distance . . . being happy to rest in the beautiful nothingness. Seeing Ben at my side . . . being thankful for his quiet . . . feeling as light as a leaf being wafted in the currents . . .

Marcia died during the middle of one cold winter night. She was at home with Dorothy and me, her husband Ben. We wished her good-bye and spread her ashes in the woods behind our house.

But we also knew her spirit continued to be with us. For a long time, Dorothy's bedtime ritual included telling Mommy about her day and listening to one of the tapes she had made for her. When I went to bed, I did the same. It helped to keep pictures of Marcia all around the house; her clothing remained in the closet, her favorite shawl draped over the living room couch. And the scent of her favorite perfume stayed nestled in her sweaters and purse.

When Dorothy turned three, she had a fine birthday. The house was decorated with multicolored streamers and balloons filled with helium. A great big birthday cake supported a one-foot-tall number 3. Six of Dorothy's friends came, along with grandparents and assorted adults. I found a magician to come by and entertain the kids with disappearing coins and even a rabbit that popped out of a hat.

And at nightfall, when it was time to go to bed, we walked up the stairs slowly, enjoying the glow after a good party, talking about Mommy and how happy she was that Dorothy had turned three. Dorothy snuggled into my neck and said she wanted her mommy to tuck her in. Before I could say anything, she caught sight of a purple balloon wafting up the stairs right behind us.

"Look, Daddy," she said, pointing at it.

Odd, I thought. *Why should this balloon be following us?*

When the balloon took a sharp left turn and came into Dorothy's room after us, my astute young daughter said, "Mommy is following us. She wants to say good night."

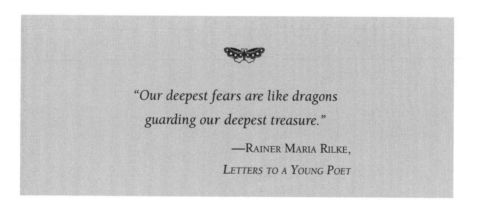

*"Our deepest fears are like dragons
guarding our deepest treasure."*

—Rainer Maria Rilke,
Letters to a Young Poet

Looking into the Mirror of Death

There's an old tale about a woman who came to see the Buddha with a dead baby in her arms. Crazed with grief, she asked for some medicine that would bring her baby back to life.

The Buddha gently offered, "There is only one way to help you. Go down to the village and bring back a mustard seed from any house in which there has been no death."

And so the woman went from house to house saying, "I have been asked by the Buddha to bring him a mustard seed from a house that has known no death."

The people in the first house said, "Many people who lived in this house died." The same was true for the second, third, and fourth houses. So it went until she had visited every house in the village. By then she realized the Buddha's request could not be fulfilled, and she brought the baby to a cemetery.

Returning to the Buddha, she explained, "I now understand your teaching. In my grief, I thought I was the only person who had ever lost a loved one. Now I remember that death visits everyone."

What fierce emotional pain the woman in this story faced, so fierce that her mind became numb. She, like many of us, found it almost impossible to accept the reality of death. The Buddha's instruction helped her understand that she wasn't alone in her misery. In one form or another, death had come to every house in the village.

Marcia felt that same fierce misery, and for a long time it numbed her mind as well. Neither she nor Ben could accept the fact of her oncoming death. It was also hard for friends and family . . . I had trouble, too. That such a young mother should die felt so wrong, so unjust, my mind refused to deal with it. All this reminded me of my son who, at age two, used to hide by turning his back to me, assuming that if he couldn't see me, I couldn't see him.

Nevertheless, for Marcia, the reality of death came ever closer. And she asked, "How can this be happening to me? And why is it happening when I have such a little baby? Have I been abandoned by God?"

Most people fell silent when they heard those questions. They didn't even know how to begin to look for such answers. Indeed, they turned to Marcia herself for help, perhaps because they sensed this was the work of the dying. Ultimately, Marcia did undertake that work. She was brave enough to seek the answers by looking *in the mirror of death*. And so she found herself in the dance of impermanence.

She saw how the tiny baby was born and grew into a magnificent infant, only to fade as the young toddler appeared. She glanced out the window of her hospital room and saw the beauty of a pink dogwood in glorious bloom and knew those blossoms would fall within a week. These are the mini-deaths that are part of life. They are also the footprints the living can follow to comprehend death.

Marcia died slowly enough to feel the young body vanish and the sick body appear, slowly enough to watch her personality itself begin to fade. And she came to understand that human beings struggle with death from the moment they're born. Recall how hard it is for a young child to move from consciousness to sleep? That's because a child doesn't have the capacity to spin a story that connects the dots of today and tomorrow, past and future, and so losing consciousness becomes a mini-death. As the child grows up she learns how to connect those dots, but usually by focusing on continuity rather than change.

As we move closer to death, we're more likely to make death another dot. Marcia was able to do that. In meditation, she could even watch her mind struggle against it. Ultimately, however, the effort became too hard, like trying to swim against a great tide, and she relaxed into it, gaining even more insight into impermanence. Looking into the mirror of death, she saw how dying opened into the larger whole. Then the loss of her physical life and even the loss of Dorothy, though terribly painful, weren't as senseless and hateful as they had once appeared.

This is a strange culture we are born into, particularly because we close our eyes to the wild and woolly nature of life. Until we're close to death, most of us persist in seeing continuity and permanence rather than the fundamental impermanence of life. We believe in a self that remains essentially the same, although it actually goes through radical mind/body transformations all through life. We aren't aware of how our bodies are changing as cells die and others take their place, nor are we aware of how our psyches are changing as experience leaves its mark. Learning to live wisely includes putting our arms around what we can interchangeably call impermanence, change, death—or life.

Lying in her bed, in the stillness that can occur during serious illness, Marcia saw how every breath arose, expanded in the body, and faded into nonexistence in time for the next breath to begin. Every moment was born, expanded, died, and was replaced by the next. Looking out the window, she gasped at the beauty of the blue sky; turning away, she realized the moment of blue sky was gone and a new moment already present. Awareness of the impermanence of life made each moment all the more precious.

I helped her with this by guiding her through meditations that revealed both the impermanence of life and the peace that can be found in larger wholes. One of those meditations was on the rising and falling away of the many bothersome sounds that hospitals produce. I recall focusing our awareness on the sounds all around us, listening to each ring of the communications system and each clang of the medical equipment until they joined together in some kind of complex orchestration. That was a larger whole. It came with a deep sense of peace. This same peace can also be found in the larger whole called the dance of life and death.

Whether or not we notice this dance of life and death depends on the way we think about ourselves, the universe, and the mystery of life and death. You might call this our *cosmology*. In Western culture, for instance, most of us have grown up with some acquaintance with the Bible, and so we understand the ancient cosmology it presents. Within this framework, we know God gives us breath at birth and takes it away at death. We are created in His likeness, but we are also mortal. For us, death is built into the divine order. And heaven or hell awaits us. All this is not for us to understand; it simply has to be. It's God's universe. He holds it in his two hands. The human being is a bystander in the divine creation. For many of us living today, this explanation is comforting; it explains the mystery of life and death in a way that satisfies and gives death a place in the human experience.

However, according to our modern way of thinking, cosmologies, like everything else, change. Historians have studied how, during the sixteenth and seventeenth centuries, a new cosmology began to take form. Science was the medium in which it took place: Galileo measured the movement of the planets, Descartes created the fundamentals of modern mathematics, and Newton conceptualized the laws of motion. In doing so, they put no authority, not even religion, above this empirical evidence. So the hold of our traditional cosmology loosened. We were no longer simply bystanders in God's universe; we were powerful players, because we had discovered certain basic laws of nature and used them to alter life.

This scientific cosmology has its problems. To the degree that we understood these universal laws, we used them to control nature, and so nature became a resource to be exploited. As we know, this path is still compelling: just open a science fiction book, and you may very well read a futuristic version of it, perhaps about a human being leaving Earth to conquer other planets.

Another problem with this cosmology is that the scientists who developed it were "materialists," which means they studied "things" in the external world. Whatever wasn't a thing, or an energy that pushed the thing, didn't exist. The cosmos they studied was inert, lifeless. So life itself became an anomaly, a miracle that was disconnected from everything else. And while death surely happened, some believed it wasn't necessary. After all, we've learned how to surpass gravity and fly through the air. Perhaps it was a mistake to make human death a part of the picture, a mistake that had to be corrected—by us. Death was disconnected from everything else—the ultimate, senseless ending.

By the time we came to the twentieth century, the universe was an empty, cold, impersonal void, sparsely strewn with molten stars, ice cold moons, and various other inert objects, and in between, in the vast stretches of space, there was nothing. The void became even more vast as astronomers trained their high-tech telescopes still farther out, and as a result human beings became infinitesimally small. We weren't even particularly special, having evolved from grubs and slime like everything else. By the new millennium, we became much like the virus or bacteria, playing out our infinitesimal and often destructive lives in a meaningless void. In fact, it appeared that we were destroying the very earth we needed to go on living.

But this cosmology also is changing. And Marcia and Ben's generation are at the forefront of that change. As members of the first generation of children to see our green planet photographed from space, they know the earth as a living organism, awesomely beautiful, alone in space, and desperately in need of our protection. This generation has begun to understand that we're all part of nature, and nature itself is alive. The vision is mesmerizing. And they want to live in resonance with it.

When I asked Marcia and Ben why they had a home birth for their child, they explained, "A home birth is healthier and more natural. We knew we might need modern medicine, and we had medical backup available, but we really wanted the baby to be born at home." So they and their midwife labored at home, in rhythm with Marcia's muscles as they tightened into hard contractions and expanded into periods of rest, creating a rhythm of expansions and contractions that resulted in Dorothy's birth.

While our traditional cosmology assumes the universe to be a fixed, unchanging background, and our scientific description sees it as inert but in motion, the new cosmology makes it organic, alive. Marcia and Ben felt they were in resonance with the rhythms of the universe as they gave birth to Dorothy.

As the couple faced Marcia's death, they shaped the experience to align with their understanding of the universe. In so doing, death was not an end but a transition from the physical to the spiritual. They didn't kill Marcia's spirit after she died but made a place for it. Marcia made audiotapes so her child could continue to feel her presence and learn how to relate to her in spirit. While the preparation of the tapes was terribly sad, it was also a highly creative effort borne of her insight into the dance of life and death.

Marcia's relationship with her mother also underwent a transformation from the physical to the spiritual. Neither woman had ever been truly happy with the other. It was a painful relationship that couldn't continue as it was. When Marcia was dying, however, she sorely missed a mother's presence. And she had the bone dream. Precious bones they were, the essence of the mother-daughter relationship. The dream was an enigma that pestered her. If only she could understand it. Then the insight came: the bag of bones held the mother love she needed! She knew this because every time she held the bag in her imagination she felt good, peaceful. Her mother was with her in the best possible way. So it was that Marcia was able to receive the gift of her mother's spirit. And she could hold that spirit in her mind whenever she wanted.

The cosmology now arising in the West is also the child of science, but, interestingly, it harkens back to the traditional cosmology as well as to ancient Eastern thought. In this new-old story, spirit enters the world again, and the universe becomes more than some combination of inert objects. The void, once thought to be empty, is alive. Zen masters call it a pregnant nothingness. In it, life is born, dies, and is born again.[1]

Here's how one interpreter of physics describes the same phenomenon in the world of subatomic particles.

> Every subatomic interaction consists of the annihilation of the original particles and the creation of new subatomic particles. The subatomic world is a continual dance of creation and annihilation, of mass changing into energy and energy changing into mass. Transient forms sparkle in and out of existence, creating a never-ending, forever newly created reality.
>
> —*Gary Zukav,* The Dancing Wu Li Masters

To know this pregnant nothingness, we need a new set of tools. Rather than the logic that worked so well in the material world of things, we listen with the third ear, rely on intuition, and wait for insight. We shift our time sense to see change happening, resonate with the ebb and flow of the tides, the rising and waning of the moon, and try to sense the flow of another human being. Everything is interconnected. Spiritual love is the energy that ties the universe together and compassion the human expression of it. This is holistic knowing. Words don't do justice to the experience; abstractions don't work. The larger whole must be experienced to be understood.[2]

We are fortunate to be living at a time when such an organic view of the universe is emerging. Many of us are participating in its creation. Therapists teach people how to listen with their third ear, use intuition, and see themselves as ever changing beings. Scientists talk about the universe as a living entity. The Internet has become a vast web of overlapping relationships, a human rendition of the larger whole. Business leaders begin to turn their focus on the importance of all the interconnections between working groups within the larger corpus.

This is important work. If enough of us participate, this view of the universe might stimulate a greater protection of the earth and all the beings on it. Marcia did her part by watching pain come and go, by seeing the magic of one moment expand and contract, and so allow for the next moment's arising. She sensed the peace that comes with silence, intuited that this was the nature of the larger whole, and felt she belonged.

How important it is to honor the process of dying! The ultimate gift we can give to ourselves and to our loved ones is to make room for their death, that process of separating the physical from the spiritual. And how much there is to learn from those who are dying! They help us know our loved ones will remain in our minds for as long as we're alive. Indeed, our relationship with the dead will change as we change, and so offer ever deepening levels of meaning.

After Marcia died, Ben and Dorothy kept Marcia alive in their house through pictures, the audiotapes, and memory. And Ben's life contracted into home and a little work. He cried a lot and spoke to the Marcia that remained in his mind and to her spirit as it infused the house. But the living carry on. Years later, when Dorothy was eight, Ben found another woman whom he and Dorothy could love, and who could love them. And Ben knew Marcia would be pleased.

The practice of meditation teaches a way of knowing. It offers a set of tools that can help us connect with the larger whole. This knowing, as all knowing, takes place through the senses. Slowing down time and observing the senses closely, we lose the focus on content. No longer does it matter what we feel or think or hear; rather, we experience the contour of feeling or the sound of thought, the energy of an emotion. This is undifferentiated or holistic knowing.

In the following meditation, we return full circle to the meditation of the very first chapter and the search for stillness. This time, however, we'll focus solely on breathing as a path toward this stillness. We'll watch body sensations associated with the breath and listen to our internal conversation. In this way, we'll examine our reactions to such a limited awareness and observe any possible resistance to it. There's a sacrifice that comes with such a laser beam attention. As you sit, you're likely to discover that it means letting go of all the tremendous attention we give to the self.

When you're ready, prepare for this last meditation by finding a quiet place to sit. Once again, read the whole meditation through once, and then follow the instructions.

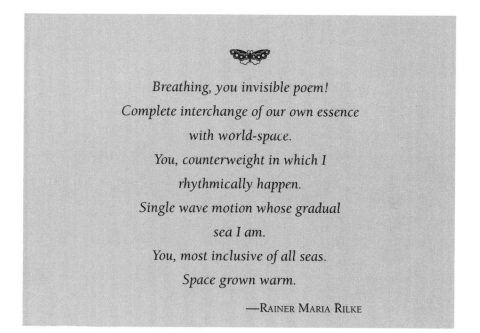

Breathing, you invisible poem!
Complete interchange of our own essence
with world-space.
You, counterweight in which I
rhythmically happen.
Single wave motion whose gradual
sea I am.
You, most inclusive of all seas.
Space grown warm.

—RAINER MARIA RILKE

A Meditation on Letting Go

Place your awareness on the body. Two arms, two legs, a torso, and a head. Drop the shoulders an inch or two . . . loosen the many small muscles around the eyes . . . the mouth . . . the jaw. Cover the whole of the body with awareness . . . its width . . . its height . . . its depth.

Gently bring your awareness to the tip of your nose. On the in-breath, feel the cool air as it enters your nostrils . . . and then sweeps past the back of your throat. Feel that same air as it leaves your body on the out-breath . . . now warm . . . so warm you can hardly detect it as it moves past the back of your throat . . . and out into the atmosphere through your nostrils. Keep your awareness on the tip of your nose and the back of your throat as the air comes in and goes out.

This isn't always easy, so try to relax into it.

As you meditate, you may be aware of being pulled into events going on around you. If that happens, simply watch how you are being pulled . . . and return to the tip of your nose and the back of your throat.

Instead, you may be pulled toward internal talk. If so, be aware . . . and gently return to the tip of your nose and the back of your throat. All is well. That's the way the mind works.

On the in-breath, feel the cool air as it enters through your nostrils and moves past the back of your throat. Feel that same air on the out-breath as it leaves your body . . . now warm . . . moving past the back of your throat and past the tip of your nose.

Take five minutes to continue this part of the meditation.

❦

Now let your awareness settle on your rib cage. Note how the rib cage expands on the in-breath and contracts on the out-breath. Attend closely.

In particular, pay attention to the moment of peace after the out-breath and before the next in-breath.

Take five minutes to stay with this phase of the meditation. See if you can catch that moment of peace and relax into it.

❦

When you return, let go of the focus on the rib cage and make the object of meditation the whole body. See if you can detect the breath as broadly in the body as possible. Feel the whole body as you breathe.

Does your global experience of breath have a shape? Is it smaller or bigger than your body?

Notice any differences between the in-breath and the out-breath.

Settle in for ten minutes and keep your awareness on the whole body and the breath. Feel the waves of muscle expansions and contractions that take place as you breathe. Rest in those waves.

❦

This time, place some of your awareness on the rib cage and some on the whole body. In so doing, you can observe the breath locally as your rib cage expands on the in-breath and contracts on the out-breath. And you can observe the breath globally as it affects your whole body.

Notice any changes in the breath, either globally or locally. Is it slowing *down? Speeding up? Is there a difference in the shape of the local and global experience of breath?*

Just watch, with equanimity . . . and ride on the waves of the breath.

Take ten minutes to continue this phase of the meditation.

❀

Sit for a while longer and investigate your reactions to limiting your awareness to the breath. Was it hard to maintain your concentration? Did you feel bored? Did you feel like jumping out of your skin? Or was this meditation a pleasure? It can be any of the above. Each is grist for the mill.

If the meditation is pleasurable, continue and see what arises.

If meditating on the breath is hard, ask yourself, What am I sacrificing? How hard is it to let go of internal talk? What has to be endured?

Sit quietly for just a few minutes, and continue to be aware of your body both globally and locally as you breathe. Recall the trouble you identified in the first meditation, and experience it within the stillness. Wait for what arises.

❀

Congratulations! To come this far—through all nine meditations—takes a strong determination and a good dose of curiosity. You have now had an experience with Mindfulness Meditation and the insight it offers.

If the meditations in this book have been helpful, continue to use them. Explore the resources listed in the bibliography so that you can pursue meditation . . . in all the ways that intrigue you.

May all beings know peace.

Training for Awareness

1. Be aware of the tip of your nose and the back of your throat as you feel the air move in and out of your body.

2. Be aware of your rib cage as you breathe in and out.

3. Be aware of the whole body as you breathe in and out.

4. Be aware of the whole body and your rib cage as you breathe in and out.

Epilogue

Now that the stories are told and the meditations ended, it's time to say good-bye. Maybe the best way to do that is to think about what lingers after all the pages have been turned.

For me, it's Tanya's song—and how she came out of her deep grieving with the urge to sing the blues. It's Nancy's healing—and how she transformed a so-called mental illness into a way of listening for those truths that lie beyond reason. And in the last story, it's Marcia's dying—and how she followed a spiritual path toward death.

I'll never forget the power of the phrase "You're a jewel, Laura. Trust in that and let yourself shine," which resounded in Laura's mind as she faced the shame that arose with her attraction to women. And in Kate's story, what stands out is the *NO* that she heard inside when her abusive husband came to the door. Maria's story about the horrors of incest has always distressed me. But what better gift on the path than a beautiful baby named Maria, for a mother who thought herself a whore?

Imprinted in my mind is also the image of Mae, the foster care mother, standing on the kitchen table with a butterfly net in her hand trying to catch a yellow canary while three children were babbling below and chocolate chip cookies were about to burn in the oven. In one form or another all mothers know this experience—along with the feeling of being overwhelmed that comes with it. Last, Harriet's once-a-year visit to Savannah to see her childhood boyfriend lives in my memory as a rite of spring. All these women found themselves in archetypical experiences, and as they faced them, they created a legacy for the rest of us.

What continues to linger in *your* memory about these stories? If you like, take a moment to recall phrases, visualize images, or even access feelings in your body that may have arisen as you read. It's a way of completing the book for yourself.

Each of the women developed the power, the fire inside, that's needed to deeply engage in great trouble. When the fire got hot enough, something inside broke, and all their fixed beliefs, the repetitive thoughts by which they shaped their lives, lost their energy—at least for a while. These were the moments when they gained insight into the larger whole. Examining the stories of these eight women, we can see the process.

Sweet are the uses of adversity
Which, like the toad, ugly and venomous,
Wears yet a precious jewel in his head;
And this our life, exempt from public haunt,
Finds tongues in trees, books in the running brooks,
Sermons in stones, and good in everything.

—WILLIAM SHAKESPEARE

NAMING TROUBLE

Given a name, trouble is no longer a secret that's hidden even from oneself. Naming can be remarkably helpful. Just think of the relief Maria felt when she realized she was a survivor of incest—as was the woman with whom she was having lunch.

NAMING THE EMOTIONS THAT ACCOMPANY TROUBLE

Anger, sadness, and fear are the emotions people most often bring to therapy. In my experience, shame and embarrassment come next. These emotions can keep us so submerged in ourselves that we can't get free of them. What a delight when interest, excitement, pleasure, and joy take their place.

CULTIVATING COMPLETE ACCEPTANCE

While we might be able to name our trouble, the mind often continues to fight the reality that it exists. We avoid in many ways, including having a drug or alcohol addiction or perhaps by engaging in indiscriminate sex. Some people live their entire lives in this avoidance. Others finally know the moment when the mind bottoms out long enough to be open to the *is-ness* of trouble—be it the loss of a loved one, the fear of going crazy, or the horror of incest. When Maria realized that no amount of sex would heal her loneliness and no amount of self-blame would make the incest go away, she was bewildered. She didn't know what to do. But she did know there was no way out; she simply had to accept the reality of her past, and it had profoundly affected her entire mind/body process.

Accepting the is-ness of our *emotions* is as important as accepting the is-ness of *trouble*. This is not an easy task for most people, especially when it comes to emotions like rage and shame. It was hard for Laura, the woman who was attracted to women, to accept the reality that shame was driving her life. It threatened to undermine her sense of herself as a free soul. Ultimately, she understood that her deep acceptance of shame led to greater freedom.

DEVELOPING EQUANIMITY

Healing calls for a special state of mind—a stillness, a patience, an impartiality that comes when we move beyond right and wrong. To cultivate this state of mind, we breathe spirit into our being, in this way touching the larger whole. Then it's possible to invite our monsters into the kitchen, offer them a cup of tea, and make friends with them.

EXPLORING THE MIND/BODY PROCESS

To heal, we need to know our internal monsters fully, completely. In the language of Mindfulness Meditation, this means developing the equanimity with which we can first locate our troublesome emotions. No doubt, they're in the *body*. So we ask many questions, such as *Does something hurt? Are there tears? How does it feel to take a deep breath?* Then we look to the *mind* and ask questions such as *How often does blame arise? Is there confusion? How hard is it to remember that the problem even exists?* Last, we also look for our emotions in the *images* we produce. *Are there images that repeat themselves in dreams or fantasies? Do they come with thoughts? Do they come with feelings in the body?* This is the process we use, and the aim is to know our monsters as fully as possible.

FORMING AN OBSERVING SELF

All this work we do in Mindfulness Psychotherapy strengthens the muscle of the observing self. It's a tool for leading the examined life and, paradoxically, a way to let go of the preoccupation with self. The more we observe, the more we become aware of the impermanence of the self.

PRACTICING COMPASSION

All the women in *Emotional Healing through Mindfulness Meditation* learned to explore the equality of compassion to help themselves heal. Sometimes they consciously practiced it with forethought by bringing loving kindness into their lives. At other times they didn't have to make compassion happen; rather, it bubbled up naturally. Mae offers an example. Becoming aware of her anger at the foster children, she discovered that it hid shame and a sense of inadequacy. Truth be told, she wasn't as good at being a foster mother as she claimed. And because her anger was used to hide her feeling of inadequacy, it wasn't as much of a strength as she thought. These insights were profound. Something inside broke. Strangely enough, being broken was exhilarating! It came with a surge of compassion for herself and her foster children. Indeed, she felt it for all the parents and all the children in the foster care system. Now she knew the is-ness of both her anger *and* her compassion.

This is a good moment to understand that each story in this book is but one chapter in a woman's life. There are and will be still other chapters. By now, the triumphs that took place are likely to have found their way into daily life; that, at least, is the goal of Mindfulness Psychotherapy. It's also likely that each woman has already revisited, or will revisit, some new rendition of her trouble. This is still another opportunity for healing—and another step along the path toward wholeness. Having triumphed once, it's more likely each woman will do so again.

Now we're back full circle to the *experience of wholeness* with which this epilogue began. That experience led to Tanya's song, Nancy's capacity to heal, and Marcia's spiritual path toward death. Eastern wisdom teaches that we don't make such experiences happen; instead, we *receive* them as insights into the unbroken fullness of the larger whole. Those moments are transforming, enlightening. They stay in our minds forever.

On the other hand, Western wisdom teaches that we can *make* the experience of wholeness happen; with the right technique and enough effort, insights or even enlightenment will arise. We tend to believe we can intentionally *devise* this technique, *design* this practice, and *create* a process that will work. As you can see, verbs take the place of nouns in our thinking, and so the Eastern *path toward wholeness* becomes the Western effort *to know holistically*.

I believe that both Eastern and Western wisdom have a place in our search for wholeness. We can wait patiently, with awareness and equanimity, for the insights that lead to transformation, and in addition, we can actively work to create the conditions within which these insights will arise. Indeed, Mindfulness Psychotherapy teaches both. We learn how to know holistically by bringing mindfulness and equanimity to our trouble, and then we wait for the insight and transformation that will naturally bubble up. In effect, we learn how to actively create the context within which we can patiently wait.

And there are many different contexts within which we can wait. Some people experience holistic knowing through music or art. I have a friend who paddles his canoe out on a river well before dawn to place himself within the magic of a sunrise—all in preparation for holistic knowing. And others immerse themselves in physical activity to do the same. The

Japanese, in particular, have been adept in creating contexts within which holistic knowing is actually a requirement. The tea ceremony is one, the physical act of writing another, and haiku poetry a third.

You might then ask, *How will I recognize holistic knowing? What exactly is it?* I offer you my limited understanding of that experience.

- Holistic knowing is an aesthetic experience. Whether in the form of deep stillness, radiant light, great clarity, or richly enhanced colors, everything manifests in great beauty. Harriet, the woman who found her childhood lover, described a few brief moments of holistic knowing after they were intimate. In that knowing, the sky became stunningly blue; indeed, everything around her was saturated with a depth of color that was more beautiful than seemed possible. Such is the aesthetic experience during an experience of holistic knowing. It's possible to experience the same intensity as a feeling of great peace, heightened exhilaration, or remarkable joy. A friend talked about the welling up of exhilaration as she walked through woods in an early morning haze and felt immersed in the whole of the scene. Knowing such a woodland holistically is a spiritual experience.

- Holistic knowing takes place in a realm that's beyond distinctions, whether they be distinctions of inside and outside, before and after, self and other, or good and bad. It's a realm where we inter-are, everything is of equal value, and it all fits together in a seamless whole. The poet Rumi wrote about this realm using a few very simple words: "Out beyond wrong-doing and right-doing lies a field. I'll meet you there."

- Holistic knowing tends to emerge in the midst of what we think of as chaos. Interestingly, this is just what makes us uncomfortable. If it happens that we find ourselves in the midst of chaos, we tend to work very hard to create the order that will reduce our discomfort. So we sort things, separate the so-called significant from the insignificant, add and subtract, divide and conquer, and look for organizing principles. In effect, we use our rational minds to figure things out.

As it turns out, this is exactly the opposite of the skills we need in order to know holistically. Instead, we need the patience to live within chaos, the capacity to manage the anxiety that arises, and the courage to explore another way of knowing. Doing this, we're likely to see the patterns that emerge in chaos. That's when the world, and everything within it, becomes an interconnected whole. Albert Einstein once said, "The intuitive mind is a sacred gift and the rational mind is a faithful servant. We have created a society that honors the servant and has forgotten the gift."

- Holistic knowing takes place beyond words—not only the words we use to make sense of chaos, but also the words that keep filling up our minds, whether they're strung together to create judgments or fantasies, whether we use them to plan for the future or to reconstruct the past. In all these ways, words themselves stop us from being here, where we are, now. Carlos Castaneda's shamanic guide, Don Juan, once said, "A man or woman of knowledge is aware that the world will change completely as soon as they stop talking to themselves."

- Last, out of the depths of holistic knowing comes love, whether in the form of compassion, generosity, or loving kindness. The miracle is that we don't have to create that love because the seeds of it are already within us. Those seeds grow luxuriously when we live within the realm of holistic knowing. In the words of a fourteenth-century English country parson, the holistic knowing of God (or the larger whole) occurs when we are *one'd with* by love. According to this spiritual insight, holistic knowing is *being* love.

Being as it is,
What's that?
In a waterdrop
Shaken from a crane's beak:
An image of the moon.

—DOGEN

I found an interesting effort to explain holistic knowing in *The Embodied Mind* by Varela, Thompson, and Rosch: "It is as if one were born already knowing how to play the violin and had to practice with great exertion only to remove habits that prevented one from displaying that virtuosity."[1]

May all beings know holistically.

Notes

For full bibliographical information on the works cited here, see the bibliography.

Dedication

The quoted material on the dedication page is from Rainer Maria Rilke, *Letters to a Young Poet*, 59.

Introduction

1. The list of written material that touches on the relationship between Buddhist meditation and psychotherapy is long. The following books have informed my thinking:

   Mark Epstein, *Going To Pieces While Falling Apart.*

   ———, *Thoughts Without a Thinker.*

   Eric Fromm, D. T. Suzuki, and Richard DeMartino, *Zen Buddhism and Psychoanalysis.*

   Robert Rosenbaum, *Zen and the Heart of Psychotherapy.*

   John Welwood, *Toward a Psychology of Awakening.*

2. Mindfulness or Insight Meditation is defined and described by Shinzen Young in these paragraphs. See:

   Shinzen Young, *Purpose and Method of Vipassana Meditation.*

3. On naming and accepting the reality of trouble, see:

   Thich Nhat Hanh, *The Heart of the Buddha's Teaching*.

4. For audiotapes of Shinzen Young's meditations, see his Web site, www.shinzen.org. You can reach him by e-mail at VSI@grte.net. Or write to The Vipassana Support Institute, 4070 Albright Avenue, Los Angeles, California 90066, for the following:

   Shinzen Young, *A Complete Guide to the Core Practice*.

5. Other references on Mindfulness Meditation:

   Stephen Batchelor, *Buddhism Without Beliefs*.

   Joko Beck, *Nothing Special*.

   Joseph Goldstein, *The Experience of Insight*.

   ———, *Insight Meditation*.

   Thich Nhat Hanh, *The Heart of the Buddha's Teaching*.

   ———, *Interbeing*.

   ———, *The Miracle of Mindfulness*.

   ———, *Thundering Silence*.

   Ayya Khema, *Be An Island*.

   Jack Kornfield, *After the Ecstasy, the Laundry*.

   ———, *Living Dharma*.

   ———, *A Path With Heart*.

   Sogyal Rinpoche, *The Tibetan Book of Living and Dying*.

   Ajan Sumedho, *The Mind Is the Way*.

   Shunryu Suzuki, *Branching Streams Flow in the Darkness*.

   ———, *Zen Mind, Beginner's Mind*.

Chapter 1. How Tanya Found Her Song

1. The concept of a holding environment was introduced by Donald Winnicott. It is a therapeutic context that is physically and emotionally safe, that is accepting and nurturing of the person, empathic and dependable. See:

   Donald Winnicott, "The Theory of the Parent-Child Relationship," 238–39.

2. For a description of the right way to sit, see:

   Thich Nhat Hanh, *The Heart of the Buddha's Teaching*.

Chapter 2. Kate's Loving Addiction

1. Martin Buber, *I and Thou*.

2. Much has been written about awareness: the continuum of awareness, choiceless awareness, one-pointed awareness. I refer you to:

   Joko Beck, *Nothing Special*.

   Pema Chodron, *The Wisdom of No Escape*.

   Rabbi David A. Cooper, *God Is a Verb*, 34.

   Thich Nhat Hanh, *The Heart of the Buddha's Teaching*.

   Stephen Levine, *A Gradual Awakening*, 17–31.

3. Shinzen Young, *A Complete Guide to the Core Practice*.

Chapter 3. Sex, Fantasy, and a Married Woman Named Laura

1. There have been many renditions of this idea of multiple selves. See:

   M. Foucault, *Madness and Civilization*.

   ———, *Mental Illness and Psychology*.

   James M. Glass, *Shattered Selves*.

   Walt Whitman, *Leaves of Grass*.

   Last, in Buddhism, the concept called impermanence implies the ever changing nature of all phenomena, including the self. Of course, the Buddhists go one step further and say that the self, if watched closely enough, disappears as a unitary phenomena. See:

   Thich Nhat Hanh, *The Heart of the Buddha's Teaching*.

2. On selfing, see:

   Rabbi David A. Cooper, *God Is a Verb*, 69–72.

3. Placing the sound of the internal voice where it is usually experienced, in the head and between the two ears, helps the meditator focus. See:

   Shinzen Young, *A Complete Guide to the Core Practice*.

Chapter 4. Maria

1. On narcissism: Many people have relationships that leave them feeling alienated and untrue to themselves. Psychotherapists assume this is be-

cause they grew up with a parent who was too self-absorbed or narcissistic to give them the attention, the recognition, or (to use a word introduced by Heinz Kohut) the *mirroring* needed for a healthy self. Buddhists believe it's craving, aversion, and ignorance that causes narcissism. For psychotherapists and Buddhists, freedom from narcissism comes with exposing and examining whatever this self is or is not. For psychotherapists it leads to a more authentic self. For Buddhists, this exposure is a first step toward letting go of the self, accepting its impermanence, and taking the path toward a spiritual life. See:

> Mark Epstein, *Thoughts Without a Thinker.*

> Heinz Kohut, *Self Psychology and the Humanities.*

2. The false self is described by Donald Winnicott as "a front to cope with the world . . . a defense to protect the true self." See:

> Donald Winnicott, *Home Is Where We Start From,* 33.

3. To read more about the problem of the self, see:

> Thich Nhat Hanh, *The Heart of the Buddha's Teaching,* 133–36.

> John Welwood, *Toward a Psychology of Awakening,* 35–47.

Chapter 5. How Nancy Gave Birth to a Healer

1. On DNA, see:

> National Health Museum, *The Search for DNA—The Birth of Molecular Biology.*

On black holes, see:

> James Glanz, "Evidence Points to Black Hole at the Center of the Milky Way."

On neutrinos, see:

> Lee Smolin, *The Life of the Cosmos.*

2. On Deconstructionists, see:

> M. Foucault, *Madness and Civilization.*

> ———, *Mental Illness and Psychology.*

3. On impermanence and the self, see:

> Guy Armstrong, "Am I or Am I Not?" 6.

> Stephen Batchelor, *Verses from the Center.*

> Bhikku Bodhi, translator, *The Connected Discourses of the Buddha.*

Thich Nhat Hanh, *The Diamond that Cuts Through Illusion*.

4. Rabbi David A. Cooper, *God Is a Verb*, 69–72.

5. On internal seeing read: Shinzen Young, *A Complete Guide to the Core Practice*.

Chapter 6. Strawberries

1. For a metaphor of the two disciplines that make up Mindfulness Psychotherapy, see:

    Shunryu Suzuki, *Zen Mind, Beginner's Mind*, 31.

2. For the story of peanut butter cookies and the separate self, see:

    Thich Nhat Hanh, *The Heart of the Buddha's Teaching*, 133.

3. I found the following article helpful in translating the essentially individualistic language of ancient Buddhism into the group-conscious, politically and culturally conscious language of our modern times. See:

    Ken Jones, "The Institutional I," 22.

4. On the BIT meditation, see:

    Shinzen Young, *A Complete Guide to the Core Practice*.

Chapter 7. Mae Is Changing the World

1. On compassion, see:

    Stephen Batchelor, *Buddhism Without Beliefs*, 84–90.

    Thich Nhat Hanh, *The Heart of the Buddha's Teaching*, 172–73.

    Sogyal Rinpoche, *The Tibetan Book of Living and Dying*, 187–208.

2. On interbeing, see:

    Thich Nhat Hanh, *Interbeing*.

3. On chaos theory, see:

    James Gleick, *Chaos*.

Chapter 8. Harriet's Love Story

1. On the different kinds of love, see:

    Rabbi David A. Cooper, *God Is a Verb*. This mystical interpretation of spiritual love recognizes how all love, erotic and spiritual, is interconnected.

    Thich Nhat Hanh, *Cultivating the Mind of Love*.

—————, *The Heart of the Buddha's Teaching.*

C. S. Lewis, *The Four Loves.* This analysis of love from a Christian perspective equates spiritual love with gift-love, loving kindness with friendship.

On the *I-we* polarity, see:

Barbara Miller Fishman with Laurie Ashner, *Resonance.*

Chapter 9. Marcia Wants to Live until She Dies

1. On cosmology, see:

   Lee Smolin, *The Life of the Cosmos.*

   Francisco J. Varela, Evan Thomson, and Eleanor Rosch, *The Embodied Mind.*

   Frank Wilczek, and Betsy Devine, *Longing for the Harmonies.*

   Gary Zukav, *The Dancing Wu Li Masters.*

2. On holistic knowing, see:

   Jeremy Narby, *The Cosmic Serpent.*

   Shunryu Suzuki, *Branching Streams Flow in the Darkness.*

   Varela, Thomson, and Rosch. *The Embodied Mind.*

Epilogue

1. For the quote from Rumi, see:

   The Essential Rumi, 36.

   For the quote from Carlos Castaneda, see:

   Jack Kornfield, *After the Ecstasy, the Laundry,* 36.

   For the reference to the mystical writings of a fourteenth-century English country parson, see:

   Clifton Wolters, translator, *The Cloud of Unknowing and Other Works.* These pieces were written around 1370, at about the same time that Geoffrey Chaucer wrote his Canterbury Tales. Though the author is unknown, he was probably a priest and was certainly a mystic.

   For the quote on learning to play the violin, see:

   Varela, Thomson, and Rosch, *The Embodied Mind,* 251.

Bibliography

Armstrong, Guy. "Am I or Am I Not?" *Inquiring Mind* 18, no. 1 (Fall 2001).

Bankei, Zen Master. *The Unborn: The Life and Teachings of Zen Master Bankei.* Translated by Norman Waddell. New York: North Point Press, 1984.

Batchelor, Stephen. *Buddhism Without Beliefs: A Contemporary Guide to Awakening.* New York: Riverhead Books, 1997.

———. *Verses from the Center: A Buddhist Vision of the Sublime.* New York: Riverhead Books, 2000.

Beck, Joko. *Everyday Zen: Love and Work.* San Francisco: HarperSanFrancisco, 1989.

———. *Nothing Special: Living Zen.* New York: Harper Collins, 1993.

Bhikku, Bodhi, translator. *The Connected Discourses of the Buddha: A New Translation of the Samutta Nikaya.* Boston: Wisdom Publications, 2000.

Buber, Martin. *I and Thou.* New York: Charles Scribner's Sons, 1970.

Capra, Fritjof. *The Tao of Physics: An Exploration of the Parallels between Modern Physics and Eastern Mysticism.* New York: Bantam Books, 1975.

Chodron, Pema. *When Things Fall Apart: Heart Advice for Difficult Times.* Boston: Shambhala, 1997.

———. *The Wisdom of No Escape: And the Path of Loving Kindness.* Boston: Shambhala, 1991.

Cooper, Rabbi David A. *God Is a Verb: Kabbalah and the Practice of Mystical Judaism.* New York: Riverhead Books, 1997.

de Chardin, Pierre Teilhard. *The Future of Man*. New York: Harper & Row, 1969.

Epstein, Mark. *Going To Pieces While Falling Apart: A Buddhist Perspective on Wholeness*. New York: Broadway Books, 1998.

————. *Thoughts Without a Thinker: Psychotherapy from a Buddhist Perspective*. New York: Basic Books, 1995.

Fishman, Barbara Miller, with Laurie Ashner. *Resonance: Creating a Relationship that Gives You the Intimacy and Independence You Want*. New York: HarperSanFrancisco, 1994.

Foucault, M. *Madness and Civilization*. Translated by R. Howard. New York: Random House, 1976.

————. *Mental Illness and Psychology*. Translated by A. Sheridan. New York: Harper and Row, 1976.

Fromm, Eric, D. T. Suzuki, and Richard DeMartino. *Zen Buddhism and Psychoanalysis*. New York: Harper Colophon, 1960.

Glanz, James. "Evidence Points to Black Hole at the Center of the Milky Way." *New York Times*, 6 September, 2001, Section A, p. 21.

Glass, James M. *Shattered Selves: Multiple Personality in a Postmodern World*. Ithaca, New York: Cornell University Press, 1993.

Gleick, James. *Chaos*. New York: Viking Penguin, 1987.

Goldstein, Joseph. *The Experience of Insight: A Simple and Direct Guide to Buddhist Meditation*. Boston: Shambhala, 1976.

————. *Insight Meditation: The Practice of Freedom*. Boston: Shambhala, 1993.

Hanh, Thich Nhat. *Cultivating the Mind of Love: The Practice of Looking Deeply in the Mahayana Buddhist Tradition*. Berkeley, Calif.: Parallax Press, 1996.

————. *The Diamond that Cuts Through Illusion: Commentaries on the Prajnaparamita Diamond Sutra*. Berkeley, Calif.: Parallax Press, 1992.

————. *The Heart of the Buddha's Teaching: Transforming Suffering into Peace, Joy, and Liberation*. New York: Broadway Books, 1998.

————. *The Heart of Understanding: Commentaries on the Prajnaparamita Heart Sutra*. Berkeley, Calif.: Parallax Press, 1988.

————. *Interbeing: Fourteen Guidelines for Engaged Buddhism*. Berkeley, Calif.: Parallax Press, 1989.

————. *The Miracle of Mindfulness: A Manual on Meditation*. Boston: Beacon Press, 1975.

————. *The Sun My Heart: From Mindfulness to Insight Contemplation.* Berkeley, Calif.: Parallax Press, 1988.

————. *Thundering Silence: Sutra on Knowing the Better Way to Catch a Snake.* Berkeley, Calif.: Parallax Press, 1993.

————. *Zen Keys: A Guide to Zen Practice.* New York: Doubleday, 1974.

Jones, Ken. "The Institutional I." *Inquiring Mind* 18, no. 1 (Fall 2001).

Khema, Ayya. *Be an Island: The Buddhist Practice of Inner Peace.* Boston: Wisdom Publications, 1999.

————. *Being Nobody Going Nowhere: Meditations on the Buddhist Path.* Sommerville, Mass.: Wisdom Publications, 1987.

Kohut, Heinz. *Self Psychology and the Humanities: Reflections on a New Psychoanalytic Approach.* New York: W. W. Norton, 1985.

Kornfield, Jack. *After the Ecstasy, the Laundry.* New York: Bantam, 2000.

————. *Living Dharma.* Boston: Shambhala, 1996.

————. *A Path With Heart: A Path Through the Perils and Promises of Spiritual Life.* New York: Bantam, 1993.

Levine, Stephen. *A Gradual Awakening.* New York: Anchor Books, 1979.

————. *Who Dies? An Investigation of Conscious Living and Conscious Dying.* New York: Doubleday, 1982.

Lewis, C. S. *The Four Loves.* Orlando, Fla.: Harcourt Brace Jovanovich, 1960.

Mitchell, Stephen. *The Enlightened Heart.* New York: Harper & Row, 1989.

Narby, Jeremy. *The Cosmic Serpent: DNA and the Origins of Knowledge.* New York: Jeremy Tarcher/Putnam, 1998.

National Health Museum. *The Search for DNA—The Birth of Molecular Biology.* Museum publication. Washington, D.C., 1999.

Neihardt, John G. *Black Elk Speaks: Being the Life Story of a Holy Man of the Oglala Sioux.* Lincoln, Neb.: University of Nebraska Press, 1932.

Rilke, Rainer Maria. *Letters to a Young Poet.* Translated by M. D. Herter. New York: W. W. Norton, 1934.

Rosenbaum, Robert. *Zen and the Heart of Psychotherapy.* Philadelphia: Brunner Mazel, 1998.

Rumi. *The Essential Rumi.* Translated by Coleman Barks with John Moyne. San Francisco: HarperSanFrancisco, 1995.

Shah, Idries. *Tales of the Dervishes. Teaching-Stories of the Sufi Masters over the Past Thousand Years.* New York: E. P. Dutton, 1970.

Smolin, Lee. *The Life of the Cosmos.* New York: Oxford University Press, 1997.

Sogyal Rinpoche. *The Tibetan Book of Living and Dying.* San Francisco: HarperSanFrancisco, 1993.

Sumedho, Ajan. *The Mind Is the Way: Buddhist Reflections on Life.* Boston: Wisdom Publications, 1995.

Suzuki, Shunryu. *Branching Streams Flow in the Darkness: Zen Talks of the Sandokai.* Edited by Mel Weitsman and Michael Wenger. Berkeley, Calif.: University of California Press, 1999.

———. *Zen Mind, Beginner's Mind: Informal Talks on Meditation and Practice.* New York: Weatherhill, 1970.

Varela, Francisco J., Evan Thomson, and Eleanor Rosch. *The Embodied Mind: Cognitive Science and Human Experience.* Cambridge, Mass.: MIT Press, 1999.

Welwood, John. *Toward a Psychology of Awakening: Buddhism, Psychotherapy and the Path of Personal and Spiritual Transformation.* Boston: Shambhala, 2000.

Whitman, Walt. *Leaves of Grass.* New York: Bantam Books, 1983.

Wilczek, Frank, and Betsy Devine. *Longing for the Harmonies: Themes and Variations from Modern Physics.* New York: W. W. Norton, 1988.

Winnicott, Donald. *Holding and Interpretation: Fragment of an Analysis.* New York: Grove Press, 1972.

———. *Home Is Where We Start From.* New York: W. W. Norton, 1986.

———. "The Theory of the Parent-Child Relationship." *International Journal of Psychoanalysis* 43:238–39, 1960.

Wolters, Clifton, translator. *The Cloud of Unknowing and Other Works.* New York: Penguin Books, 1961.

Young, Shinzen. *A Complete Guide to the Core Practice.* Unpublished. For copies, write to the Vipassana Support Institute, 4070 Albright Avenue, Los Angeles, California 90066. More written material is available at his Web site: www.shinzen.org.

———. *Purpose and Method of Vipassana Meditation.* Unpublished.

Zukav, Gary. *The Dancing Wu Li Masters: An Overview of the New Physics.* New York: William Morrow, 1979.

I hope you have enjoyed and found value in
Emotional Healing through Mindfulness Meditation.

For queries, additional explanation, further
resources, or a course in healing emotions,
I can be reached at:
www.emotionalhealing.net
or
barbarafishman@emotionalhealing.net

Or you can reach me by mail at:

Dr. Barbara Miller Fishman
P.O. Box 2823
Bala Cynwyd, PA 19004